Suicide: Closing the Exits

Ronald V. Clarke   David Lester

Suicide:
Closing the Exits

Springer Verlag
New York Berlin Heidelberg
London Paris Tokyo Hong Kong

Ronald V. Clarke
School of Criminal Justice
Rutgers University
Newark, New Jersey 07102
USA

David Lester
Richard Stockton State College
Pomona, New Jersey 08240
USA

Library of Congress Cataloging-in-Publication Data
Clarke, R. V. G.
  Suicide: closing the exits/Ronald V. Clarke and David Lester.
    p.   cm.
  Bibliography: p.
  Includes index.
  ISBN 0-387-97004-5 (alk. paper)
    1. Suicide—Prevention. 2. Gun control. 3. Gases, Asphyxiating
and poisonous—Safety measures. I. Lester, David, 1942–
II. Title.
  [DNLM: 1. Suicide—prevention & control. HV 6545 C599s]
HV6545.C54   1988
362.2'87—dc20
DNLM/DLC   89–6366

Printed on acid-free paper

Typeset by Thomson Press (India) Ltd., New Delhi, India.
Printed and bound by Edwards Brothers, Ann Arbor, Michigan.
Printed in the United States of America.

9 8 7 6 5 4 3 2 1

ISBN 0-387-97004-5 Springer-Verlag New York Berlin Heidelberg
ISBN 3-540-97004-5 Springer-Verlag Berlin Heidelberg New York

Résumé

Razors pain you;
Rivers are damp;
Acids stain you;
And drugs cause cramp;
Guns aren't lawful;
Nooses give;
Gas smells awful;
You might as well live.

Dorothy Parker, 1926

Preface

This book reports a program of research concerned with the possibility of preventing suicide by restricting access to lethal agents, such as guns, drugs, and carbon monoxide. To many people, it may seem implausible that deeply unhappy people could be prevented from killing themselves by "closing the exits," but the suggestion is by no means a new one and has been current in the journals for some time. This book is the first major exposition of the idea, however, with the evidence collected in one place and an examination of the implications for understanding the suicidal person and for preventing suicide. We hope to convince public health officials that, although the idea is largely disregarded at present, restricting access to lethal agents should take its place as a major preventive strategy along with the psychiatric treatment of depressed and suicidal individuals and the establishment of suicide prevention centers in communities to counsel those who are suicidal or in crisis.

We came to this position by two different routes. R.C.'s interest derived from a concern with the role of opportunity in crime. This originated in his doctoral research dealing, not with suicide, but with another form of escape—absconding from training schools for young offenders. He found that the variance in absconding was explained more by the opportunities to abscond presented by the school's environment and regime than by the offender's history or personality. This insight influenced later research undertaken for the British government on the "situational prevention" of crime, which sought to establish that much crime can be prevented by "designing out" criminal opportunities from the environment (Clarke and Mayhew, 1980).

The main theoretical objection to this approach rests on the concept of displacement, the idea that reducing opportunities will result merely in the reappearance of crime at some other time, in some other place, or in an alternative form. While investigating this topic, R.C. came across the suggestion that the drop in the British suicide rate in the 1960s and 1970s resulted from the removal of carbon monoxide from the domestic gas supply, which rendered it nontoxic. Not only was this a striking example of the value of opportunity reduction, but, because the alternative forms of suicide are much more limited than those of crime, it also held considerable potential for the investigation of displacement. Clear documentation of the effects of gas detoxification might therefore provide strong support for situational prevention (see Clarke and Mayhew, 1988).

By contrast, most of D.L.'s professional life has been taken up with research directly concerned with suicide and its many different aspects. Prevention has been a continuing preoccupation. Following the completion of his doctoral dissertation on whether suicide can be considered an aggressive act, he worked for two years in a suicide prevention center. This led him to undertake a series of studies on the effectiveness of these centers that suggested they were generally failing in their objectives. Because of theoretical links between suicide and homicide (Henry and Short, 1954) he had also developed an interest in the latter topic and, in the course of his readings, came across a book on gun control that contained codings of the handgun statutes of each state in the United States. He had originally planned to investigate the effect of handgun control on murder, but he included state suicide rates simply because of his major research interest. Unexpectedly, he found no support for the effects of strict handgun control statutes on murder but did find an effect on suicide.

The two of us met to discuss our common interests and noted that more of those attempting to commit suicide using car exhaust were being rescued because of the reduced toxicity of car exhaust. The result was a collaborative effort to document the effects of emission controls on cars on suicidal behavior.

The stimulus of this collaborative research also pushed each of us into the other's terrain; R.C. conducted a study of firearms and suicide while D.L. has looked at domestic gas and suicide. Eventually, we decided to pull together all of our studies and investigate the theoretical and public policy issues our research, both individual and collaborative, has affected. The result is the present book, in which we lay out our findings and explore the implications of the research for both understanding and preventing suicide.

Many of the studies we report were undertaken with other colleagues and have been published in journals. The full list follows, and we take this opportunity to thank the publishers for their permission to reprint material from the original articles and our collaborators for their advice and help. We also thank Pat Mayhew and Dr. Richard Seiden for their extensive comments on the draft of this book.

Studies 1 and 2 (Chapter 2) were undertaken by R.C. together with Pat Mayhew, principal research officer of the Home Office Research and Planning Unit, London, during her period spent as visiting fellow at the National Institute of Justice in Washington. Study #1 was published as Clarke, R.V., and Mayhew, P. The British gas suicide story and its criminological implications, in M. Tonry and N. Morris (eds.) *Crime and Justice*, Vol. 10, 1988 (Chicago: University of Chicago Press). Study #2 was published as Clarke, R.V., and Mayhew, P. Crime as opportunity: a note on domestic gas suicide in Britain and the Netherlands. *British Journal of Criminology*, 29, 35–46, 1989.

Study 3 (Chapter 2) was undertaken by D.L. and was presented at the 1989 meeting of the American Association of Suicidology.

Study 4 (Chapter 3) was undertaken by D.L. and Dr. Michael Frank and published as Lester, D., and Frank, M. L. The use of motor vehicle exhaust for suicide and the availability of cars. *Acta Psychiatrica Scandinavia*, 79, 238–240, 1989.

Study 5 (Chapter 3) was undertaken jointly by the authors and published as Clarke, R.V., and Lester D. Toxicity of car exhausts and opportunity for suicide: comparison between Britain and the United States. *Journal of Epidemiology and Community Health*, 41, 114–120, 1987.

Study 6 (Chapter 4) was undertaken by D.L. and published as Availability of guns and the likelihood of suicide. *Sociology and Social Research*, 71, 287–288, 1987.

Study 7 (Chapter 4) was undertaken by D.L. and published as Gun ownership and suicide in the United States. *Psychological Medicine*, in press.

Study 8 (Chapter 4) was undertaken by D.L. and published as Restricting the availability of guns as a strategy for preventing suicide. *Biology and Society*, 5, 127–129, 1988.

Study 9 (Chapter 4) was undertaken by R.C. with Dr. Peter Jones, Department of Criminal Justice, Temple University, and published as Clarke, R.V., and Jones, P. Suicide and increased availability of handguns in the United States. *Social Science and Medicine*, 28, 805–809, 1989.

Studies 10 and 11 (Chapter 5) were undertaken by D.L. and Dr. Mary Murrell and published in Lester, D. *Gun Control: Issues and Answers.* Springfield, IL: Charles C Thomas, 1984.

Study 12 (Chapter 5) was undertaken by D.L. and published as An availability–acceptability theory of suicide. *Activitas Nervosa Superior*, 29, 164–166, 1987.

Study 13 (Chapter 7) was undertaken by D.L. and published as The perception of different methods of suicide. *Journal of General Psychology*, 115, 215–217, 1988.

Study 14 (Chapter 7) was undertaken by D.L. and published as Why do people choose particular methods for suicide? *Activitas Nervosa Superior*, 30, 312–314, 1988.

We are also grateful for permission to reproduce "Résumé" from *The Portable Dorothy Parker* and the extract from John MacDonald's novel reproduced at the beginning of Chapter 6.

Finally, all of this research, which consists of analysis of available data, required no grant support. However, we are grateful to our respective institutions for the facilities afforded us in completing this work.

Ronald Clarke
David Lester

Contents

1

Preventing Suicide

Suicide prevention is one of the major goals today of the Public Health Service of the U.S. government; indeed, this has been the case since the 1960s when the National Institute of Mental Health established a center for the study and prevention of suicide. However, as noted a few years ago in a *New England Journal of Medicine* editorial (Hudgens, 1983), the accumulation of knowledge about suicidal behavior in the last quarter of a century has failed to bring about a reduction of suicide in America.

That editorial saw three promising strategies for prevention: improvements in diagnosing and treating depression, growth of suicide prevention and crisis intervention centers, and restriction of access to lethal means for committing suicide. In this book we argue that the latter approach has not been seriously considered hitherto and that reducing access to lethal agents such as guns, drugs, and carbon monoxide has great life-saving potential. As well as reviewing existing research, we present a number of supportive studies, which use data from America and elsewhere, concerning the relationship between rates of suicide and a variety of lethal agents.

The Nature of the Problem

The suicide rates for the United States (per 100,000 of the population) during the past fifty years, presented here, indicate that suicide rates have not changed much since the Second World War, although they are lower than those of 1933 (the first year in which all states reported):

1933	15.9
1940	14.4
1950	11.4
1960	10.6
1970	11.6
1980	11.9
1985	12.3

In America in 1985, there were 29,543 suicides out of 2,086,440 deaths. It has long been known that suicide rates are higher in men than in women, in whites than in blacks, and in Native Americans than in others (Lester, 1983). However, two important features of suicide have called for special attention in the 1980s. First, rates of suicide are high among the elderly. For example in 1985, the suicide rates by age were as follows:

Age (Years)	Men	Women
10–14	2.3	0.9
15–19	16.0	3.7
20–24	26.2	4.9
25–29	25.3	5.6
30–34	23.5	6.3
35–39	22.2	6.5
40–44	22.3	7.8
45–49	23.0	8.4
50–54	24.0	8.1
55–59	26.8	8.2
60–64	26.8	7.2
65–69	29.0	6.7
70–74	38.9	7.2
75–79	48.4	7.4
80–84	61.9	6.0
85+	55.4	4.6

These figures clearly show that suicide is a major problem for those concerned with the psychological health and social well-being of the elderly, especially older men.

Second, there has been a marked increased in the suicide rates of young adults in recent years, especially among white males. The suicide rate of white males aged 15 to 19 years has risen from 9.3 in 1970 to 15.0 in 1980 (Centers for Disease Control, 1986). For white males aged 20 to 24, the rate has risen from 19.2 to 27.8 in the same period.

This increasing rate of suicide among the young has given rise to much concerned comment. Blum (1987) noted that adolescents are the only group who have not experienced improvement in their health status in the last 30 years. Death from violence has now replaced communicable diseases as the primary cause of adolescent mortality, and more than three-quarters of adolescent deaths are from suicide, homicide, and accidents. The young not only have much potential, but their recent improved material well-being makes their self-destructive tendencies hard to comprehend (Uhlenberg and Eggebeen, 1986).

Although suicide is considered a major mental health problem in America, the size of the problem is much greater in some other nations. In 1980, Hungary led the world with a rate of 45.0, almost four times the American rate. Sri Lanka had a rate of 29.2, Denmark 29.1, Austria 26.0, and Finland

and Switzerland both 24.7. Furthermore, Lester (1988d) has shown that nations with the highest suicide rates in 1970 experienced the greatest increase from 1970 to 1980. So the problem is getting worse for these nations.

The rising youth suicide rates of the United States are also found in other nations of the world. The United States had a 40 percent increase in the youth suicide rate from 1970 to 1980; Norway experienced a 224 percent increase, Spain a 93 percent increase, Switzerland an 80 percent increase, and Thailand a 78 percent increase (Lester, 1988e).

Increased suicide rates with increasing age are also found in many other nations. For example, although the overall suicide rate in Hungary in 1980 was 45.0, the rate for males over the age of 75 was 202.2, more than four times higher.

However, figures for completed suicide are but the "tip of the iceberg," for many more nonfatal suicide attempts occur than acts of completed suicide. These attempted suicides are sometimes called parasuicides, or acts of deliberate self-harm, to distinguish them from completed suicides. Many attempted suicides do not harm themselves sufficiently to come to the attention of the authorities, but it has been estimated that, for every completed suicide, there may be 8 (Farberow and Shneidman, 1961) or even 20 (Wells, 1981) attempted suicides. About 15 percent of these attempted suicides subsequently complete suicide compared with only 1 percent of the general population, so they constitute a high-risk population. One can see, therefore, that the problem of suicide is far greater than a cursory examination of rates of completed suicide might lead us to believe.

Research into the causation of suicide can be divided into psychologically inclined and sociologically inclined studies. In the psychological study of suicide, investigators have identified psychiatric disturbance, depression in particular, as the strongest indicator of a high suicidal risk. Beck and his associates have suggested that one of the cognitive components of depression, namely, hopelessness, is especially useful in predicting future suicidal actions (Beck et al., 1975).

In addition, it has frequently been noted that other types of self-destructive behaviors, such as alcoholism and drug abuse, are associated with an increased likelihood of suicide, and that stress, too (from loss of significant others, health, or status), appears to be especially great in the months before a suicide (Paykel, 1979).

Sociologically, weakened social integration and social regulation appear to be related to high rates of suicide, just as Durkheim (1897) first argued. Sociologists have found that high rates of divorce in a culture, high rates of interdistrict migration, and low rates of church attendance all are strongly associated with high rates of suicide.[1]

---

[1] The extensive research literature on suicide has been reviewed by Lester (1972a, 1983).

However, the *New England Journal of Medicine* editorial mentioned earlier was correct in arguing that the vast increase in our knowledge about suicide appears to have had few preventive benefits. And this is not through lack of communication. In the 1960s, about 1000 scholarly articles and books on suicide were published, in the 1970s about 2000, and in the 1980s about 3000 items will have appeared. Scholars are certainly writing about suicide!

Strategies for Preventing Suicide

Two major propositions are advanced in this book: that the availability of methods for committing suicide plays a causal role in suicide and that suicide can be prevented by reducing access to these methods. Before presenting the evidence for these propositions, we review the two main strategies that have been taken in the past to prevent suicide. This will facilitate comparison of our proposals with these earlier approaches, which consist of

1. establishing community suicide prevention centers *and*
2. searching for effective treatment of depressed and suicidal patients by the psychiatric and counseling professions.

Suicide Prevention Centers

Following the lead of the Los Angeles suicide clinic established in the 1950s by Edwin Shneidman and Norman Farberow, and stimulated by the National Institute of Mental Health's center for suicide prevention, communities across America established suicide prevention centers in the following decades. In the United Kingdom, the Salvation Army started an early suicide prevention service in 1905, but more recently one central organization, the Samaritans, has organized centers throughout the country.

Suicide prevention centers are primarily oriented around a crisis model of the suicidal process. People who are suicidal are conceptualized as being in a time-limited crisis state. Immediate crisis counseling is intended to help the suicidal individual through the suicidal crisis, whereupon a normal life may resume.

The centers typically operate a 24-hour telephone service that people in distress can call to talk to a counselor. Counselors are typically paraprofessionals—ordinary people who have graduated from a brief training program and use crisis intervention as the mode of counseling (active listening, assessment of resources, and problem-solving). Some centers have walk-in clinics, and a few have set up "stores" in the poorer sections of cities and crisis teams who can visit distressed people in their own homes.

The centers are well equipped for early intervention with people on the verge of suicide, but, as noted (Lester, 1972b), their approach is essentially passive. The suicidal person has to contact the center. Active approaches, such as seeking out discharged psychiatric patients, elderly males living alone, and other high-risk groups are rarely pursued. In addition, community workers such as police officers, clergy, physicians, and even groups such as bartenders, prostitutes, and hair dressers who also come into contact with the public, have rarely been sensitized to the detection of depressed, disturbed, and suicidal people so that they could refer them to suicide prevention centers.

Several studies have been done on the effectiveness of the centers. In the first, Bagley (1968) compared English cities and found that those with a suicide prevention center did have a lower suicide rate compared with cities without such a center. In a more carefully controlled study, however, Barraclough and his colleagues (Barraclough et al., 1977; Jennings et al., 1978) compared another group of English cities, matching them for ecological similarity, and found no effect of the centers on the suicide rate. Furthermore, as a result of reanalyzing Bagley's data, Lester (1980) concluded that Bagley had not in fact demonstrated the preventive effect of the centers he claimed.

Nor was much evidence of success found in a series of similar studies undertaken in the United States. Lester (1973a, 1973b, 1974a, 1974b) studied large samples of American cities, controlling for size of the city, and found no effect of centers on the suicide rate. For example, from 1960 to 1970, the suicide rate in cities without a suicide prevention center rose from 9.4 to 10.7 while the suicide rate in cities with centers rose from 12.1 to 13.6.

Bridge et al. (1977), who explored correlates of the suicide rates of 100 counties in North Carolina, found no association with the presence of a center. Because they did not examine changes in the suicide rate of the counties over time, however, their study was less than adequate. Indeed, all of the evaluations of suicide prevention centers were severely criticized by Auerbach and Kilmann (1977), who noted the impracticality of using suicide rates as a measure of effectiveness and the absence of work on treatment processes amd client behavior change.

A number of attempts were made in the 1970s to improve the work of suicide prevention centers (Resnick and Hathorne, 1973). The importance of identifying and locating high-risk groups in the population and fashioning specific programs for them was stressed. On the whole, the focus was on better ways of intervening rather than on programs to improve the social environment and thus reduce the forces leading to suicide.

One relevant study was conducted by Wold and Litman (1973), who had the excellent idea of examining the records of those who had killed themselves after calling a suicide prevention center. They found inadequate counseling on the part of some of the volunteers who handled the calls. But more important, they found that the crisis counseling approach was not a suitable means of dealing with *chronic*, high suicide risk callers who needed referral to other agencies, which typically the callers did not pursue. Wold and Litman discussed the possibility of establishing programs to deal more effectively with such callers.

In the most recent evaluation, Miller et al. (1984) have reported more favorable results. They compared a sample of counties in the United States with and without suicide prevention centers and found that the centers had a beneficial impact on the suicide rates for white females younger than 24 years of age (but for no other group). This result was replicated on a new sample of counties. Since young white females are among the more frequent callers to suicide prevention centers, this result makes sense.

Thus, at the present time it seems that the previously negative conclusions about the effectiveness of suicide prevention centers may need to be modified. If Miller's results are replicated in other locales, we may conclude that suicide prevention centers do help prevent suicide in the sociodemographic groups that they most often serve.

Psychological Treatment of the Depressed and Suicidal Person

The psychiatric/psychological approach to suicide prevention is to take individual clients and identify the most effective ways of medicating or counseling them to reduce the risk of suicide. Since depression is both the most common psychiatric syndrome and the most common mood accompanying increased potential for suicide, its treatment has been the primary focus of this approach.

The majority of suicides are found to have been psychiatrically disturbed. Barraclough (1972) examined 100 cases of completed suicide and found that 64 had had depressive illnesses. Of these, 44 had previous depressive episodes, and 21 of these met strict criteria for diagnosing "recurrent affective illness." Barraclough therefore argued for good diagnostic practices and effective treatment as a way of preventing suicide.

The provision of general psychiatric services ought to assist prevention efforts. Ratcliffe (1962) noted that the change of Dingleton mental hospital in patient management from a locked-ward to an open-door system was accompanied by a drop of about 60 percent in the number of suicides in the surrounding community during the following 10 years (while the suicide rate in Scotland, as a whole, stayed constant). Ratcliffe suggested that the open-door policy had induced more of the psychiatrically disturbed citizens in the community to use the psychiatric facility. However, no such drop in the suicide rate was noted by Walk (1967) when a community mental health center was opened in Chichester, England.

Medication is another staple of treatment. Barraclough, in his study reported earlier, argued for the use of lithium for those patients who have bipolar effective disorders. Montgomery and Montgomery (1984) have recently shown that administration of flupenthixol (a depot neuroleptic) resulted in a significant decrease in suicide attempts in suicidal patients diagnosed as having a personality disorder. In contrast, neither a placebo nor Mianserin, a less toxic oral antidepressant, had a significant effect on suicidal behavior.

Effective psychotherapy may also be of benefit for potential suicides. For example, Liberman and Eckman (1981) compared the effectiveness of behavior therapy and insight-oriented therapy for repeated suicide attempters. Each program included individual, group, and family therapy components. They found that the behavior therapy program (which included training in social skills, anxiety management, family negotiation, and contingency contracting) had a more positive outcome than the insight-oriented program after both nine months and two years. However, Montgomery and Montgomery (1982) reviewed six previous studies on the effects of counseling on suicidal behavior and found that only three were adequately designed and only one of these showed counseling had a significant impact on suicidal behavior.

Thus, while medication certainly has a place in the treatment of the depressed suicidal patient, we cannot be too optimistic about the effectiveness of the other psychiatric/psychological approaches at the present time. Furthermore, these approaches are useful only for those individuals who seek out the help of clinics or private psychotherapists for their personal problems.

Other Strategies for Preventing Suicide

Before coming to our own proposals, two other prevention strategies that have attracted little attention should be mentioned for completeness. One of these is to make suicide less likely by manipulating societal approval. As suicide becomes more common, the publicity attendant on the suicidal acts and the greater likelihood of knowing suicidal relatives, friends, or colleagues increases the likelihood that we will come to view suicide as an appropriate and acceptable solution for some of life's problems. It is possible to wage a public health campaign against such acceptance of suicide. The campaign could stress the grief and suffering caused to those close to the suicide, the pain and physiological handicaps that can result from surviving a serious suicidal attempt, and moral values opposed to suicide. This approach is considered more fully in the final chapter.

The second strategy for preventing suicide is to improve the conditions in society by reducing unemployment, finding better ways to treat disorders such as alcoholism, and improving parenting skills so that we raise psychologically healthier children. Such measures should improve the quality of life and concomitantly reduce the incidence of psychological distress and responses to this distress such as crime and suicide (Stengel, 1964). Although people will always seek to improve society, Lester (1986), who has found that nations with higher quality of life have *higher* suicide rates, questions the validity of this approach.

Reducing Access to Lethal Agents

Durkheim (1897) noted wide local or national variations in preferred methods of death. Such variations, which seem to reflect differential availability of methods or different traditions in their use, have been regularly reported in the literature ever since. For example, at the local level, Drinker (1938) reports that formerly more people in upstate New York than in New York City killed themselves with car exhaust, possibly because more upstate inhabitants had access to garages. And Seiden (1977) has shown that jumping from a high place—the Golden Gate Bridge—is a particularly common form of suicide in San Francisco, where the local byword is that, when stress gets too great, one can always "go off the bridge" (Seiden and Spence, 1983–1984).

At a national level, the high rate of suicides by gun in Australia and the United States (particularly in the southern states) has been blamed on the more widespread ownership of firearms and the development of a "gun culture" (Marks and Stokes, 1976). The most common form of suicide in the Netherlands, until 1967 (when it was replaced by barbiturate deaths), was drowning (Noomen, 1975). In India, Sri Lanka, and Malaysia, the common mode for suicide is by swallowing insecticides (usually organophosphorus compounds), which are cheap and easily available (Rao, 1975; Maniam, 1988; Berger, 1988). Berger reports: "Almost every rural grocery store has shelves full of many brands of pesticides in bottles of various sizes. Over 100 chemicals—including malathion in more than 200 formulations—are sold. Liquid preparations of pesticides can be lethal in minute doses" (p. 827). In Colombo 53 percent of suicides used pesticides, and "the proportion would be higher in agricultural areas where pesticides are even more widely available" (p. 826).

Despite the frequency of such observations, these differences have rarely been carefully studied (one notable exception discussed later is Farmer and Rohde's [1980] international comparative study), and their preventive implications have been neglected. This neglect derives from the assumption (which we believe to be mistaken) that methods of suicide can be readily substituted for one another and that deliberately restricting the availability of particular lethal agents makes little sense.

Opinions, however, seem to be changing now—largely as the result of accumulated research showing that changes over time in the use of particular methods appear to be related to their changed availability. For example, suicide by car exhaust gases have become less common in the United States as a result of emission controls (Landers, 1981; Hay and Bornstein, 1984), which have reduced the carbon monoxide concentrations in the exhaust gases of General Motors' cars, for example, from 8.5 percent in 1968 to 0.05 percent in 1980. In Britain, on the other hand, where emission controls have yet to be introduced, this form of suicide has increased in recent years, presumably as a result of increased car ownership and more widespread knowledge of this means of death (Bulusu and Alderson, 1984). It has been claimed that suicide by jumping from tall buildings increased both in Helsinki (Achte and Lonnqvist, 1975) and Taiwan (Rin, 1975) as more high buildings were built. In Britain (Adelstein and Mardon, 1975), Australia (Stoller, 1969; Whitlock, 1975), and elsewhere suicides by overdosing with barbiturates became common with the increasing prescribing of these drugs. Similarly, these suicides decreased with wider knowledge of the dangers of overprescribing—in some cases accompanied by legislation limiting their prescription—and with the availability of safer alternatives.

Perhaps the best known example of this kind, however, is the reduction in both gas suicides and the overall suicide rate following the detoxification of domestic gas in the United Kingdom (Kreitman, 1976; Brown, 1979), which is discussed at length in Chapter 2.

It is now therefore being increasingly suggested that suicide might be prevented by the removal of lethal agents from the environment of the suicidal person. Robin and Freeman-Browne (1968) noted that the majority of attempted suicides are released into home environments where lethal quantities of drugs exist, and Friedman (1966) has described cases in which patients have forged prescriptions to obtain drugs to kill themselves. Barraclough et al. (1971) recommended reductions in the size and number of prescriptions, wrapping the tablets in foil or plastic blisters, use of nonbarbiturates when possible, recalling unused tablets, setting up procedures to prevent forging of prescriptions, and not prescribing for patients without seeing them.[2] Local campaigns are regularly mounted for installing suicide nets on bridges or fences at other jumping spots favored by suicides,[3] while studies suggesting an increased role in suicide of firearms, especially among the young (Boor, 1981; Boyd, 1983), have been followed by calls for gun controls (e.g., Westermeyer, 1984).

---

[2] The following is a typical case of suicide reported by Barraclough et al. (1971) and illustrates that making large quantities of a medication available to a patient without adequate supervision facilitates the accumulation of lethal quantities, which may be used to commit suicide:

A 45-year-old, single woman lived alone since the recent death of both parents. She was drawing sick benefits on psychiatric grounds but was actively looking for work. In the preceding seven years there had been four admissions for agitated depression, with reasonable response to treatment. At the time of death the drug treatment was amitriptyline 100 mg daily and Sodium Amytal 1 G (15 gr) daily. This prescribing was recorded for the previous six months but had probably been going on for 12 months. She had not seen the doctor for seven months and obtained prescriptions on request from his receptionist. There had been a recent occurrence of her depressive symptoms. (Barraclough et al., 1971, p. 652)

[3] Recent examples are the Duke Ellington Bridge in Washington (*The Washington Post*, December 18, 1985) and the Mid-Hudson Bridge (Moss, 1986).

The Research Plan

This book presents a series of studies we have undertaken to explore the idea that deliberately restricting the availability of particular lethal agents may be an effective means of reducing suicide. It is, of course, difficult, if not impossible, to conduct experimental studies of whether the increased availability of a method for suicide leads to an increase in the use of that method for suicide and an increase in the overall suicide rate. It is not possible (or ethical) for the experimenter to manipulate an independent variable such as the availability of methods for suicide simply to see whether this affects the incidence of suicide.

However, it is possible to exploit the "natural experiments" presented by the *regional* differences mentioned previously in the availability of particular methods for suicide (for example, in the ownership of firearms) as well as by the changes that take place in the availability of a method for suicide over *time* (often without any deliberate intent to affect the incidence of suicide) to test the hypothesis in a correlational study.

In the research described in this book, we have taken advantage of some regional variations in the availability of methods for suicide to see whether these variations are related to the suicide rate. In addition, we have also identified several changes in the availability of methods for suicide over time, and we have studied the impact of these changes on the suicide rate. Although our presentation of the research is organized into a coherent order, in fact it depended to a large extent on our serendipitous discovery of such regional and temporal variations.

Previous discussion of the central hypothesis of this volume has been limited by the narrowness of the investigations. For example, Oliver and Hetzel (1972) showed that restricting prescriptions for hypnotic-strength sedatives in 1967 in Australia was followed by a drop in their use as a means of suicide. However, Gibbs and Arnold (1972) objected that the drop in the suicide rate from overdoses could have been a result of the increased availability of effective antidepressants, increases in admissions to psychiatric hospitals, and increased skill in intensive care units.

Objections can usually be made, like those of Gibbs and Arnold, to a specific time series analysis in which restriction of a particular method for suicide was accompanied by a parallel decrease in the suicide rate using that method. In this volume we show that a change in suicide over time, as one particular method for suicide becomes more or less available, can be documented in relation to three lethal agents: firearms, toxic car exhaust, and toxic domestic gas. We believe objections that can be made to the time-series analysis for one particular mode of suicide are unlikely to apply to the time series for other methods. This means that, without an alternative general hypothesis to account for our results, critics of the idea that restricting the availability of methods for suicide would prevent suicide must resort to individual post hoc alternative explanations for each particular study.

In addition, we will also provide evidence regarding two of the methods (guns and car exhaust) that regional variations in their availability are associated with their use for suicide. Proponents of any alternative explanations for the time-series association must therefore also account for the regional variation. For example, let us assume it is being claimed that the decrease in the proportion of suicides in the United States using car exhaust is really a side effect of improved care by emergency medical teams. First, evidence would need to be provided that medical care has improved in general throughout the United States and, second, this variable would also have to account for the regional variation in the use of car exhaust as a means for suicide. In contrast to this hypothetical and undocumented alternative explanation, our studies show that the use of car exhaust for suicide is related to *both* to the availability of toxic cars over time *and* the per capita ownership of cars over regions.

The Ethics of Preventing Suicide

Perhaps one final matter we must address in this chapter is the question of whether suicide should be prevented. If it is accepted that people have the right to take their own lives, an increasingly common position and one supported by the legal system which has decriminalized suicide and clearly upheld the right to refuse treatment, what right do we have to prevent people from killing themselves?

It is important to note that a great deal of suicide prevention is passive (Lester, 1981). The suicide prevention center or the counselor waits until the suicidal person calls for help. There is no coercion of the suicidal person to call for this help. The person does so because he or she wants help. Such prevention is clearly morally correct, and to refuse to help someone who asks for help would be considered immoral.

Some suicide prevention centers are more active. They seek out attempted suicides and survivors of someone else's suicide and make themselves known to these persons. However, all they can do is say, "We are here if you need us." They have no power to coerce people into counseling.

The methods for preventing suicide that we propose in this book are more active. They seek to restrict access to methods for suicide—to fence in bridges, prescribe medications in small doses, make handguns difficult to purchase, and so on. However, aside from moral grounds, legal considerations make some of these suggestions inevitable. If we can be sued by a neighbor whose child drowns in our swimming pool which we failed to fence in, then a bridge authority can be sued for failing to install fences to prevent people from jumping to their death. Similarly, a physician who overprescribes a lethal antidepressant is open to be sued by relatives of the person who uses the medication for suicide.

Moreover, restricting access to lethal methods for suicide does not absolutely prevent someone from committing suicide. Some methods, such as hanging or drowning, will always remain accessible. It merely makes it more difficult to use particular methods.[4] This difficulty may cause the person to delay the planned suicide and, if suicide is indeed a crisis state (Kessel [1976] reports that two-thirds of 522 self-poisonings he studied in Scotland were impulsive), by the time a method for suicide is found, the person may be over the suicidal crisis.

Finally, we should note that objections to making suicide more difficult rest on a patently false proposition—that there is consensus in society about the "ideal" level of difficulty for suicide and that this roughly approximates the level that presently exists.

Conclusions

It has usually been assumed that a genuinely suicidal individual will always find a way to die. However, the precipitous decline in the British rate of suicide following the detoxification of domestic gas (which is documented in Chapter 2) strongly suggests that the considerable regional and temporal variations in methods of suicide mentioned earlier may reflect differences in the incidence of the behavior just as much as in its forms (see Farmer and Rohde, 1980). This is easier to accept if suicide is seen not simply as the result of an inexorable drive to self-extinction, but rather as the combined result of deep but possibly temporary despair, the weakening of moral restraints against the behavior, *and* the availability of a method that it not too difficult or repugnant to use.

The idea that the availability of lethal agents in the environment plays a *causal* role in suicide has been resisted in the past for three reasons:

1. it seems to trivialize the behavior and demeans the personal suffering that fuels most suicides,
2. it calls into question the role of the helping professions, especially psychiatry, in prevention and
3. it is not congruent with most theories of suicide, which tend to assume a person intent on suicide can always find a way to accomplish it.

The present volume explores the possible causal role of access to lethal agents more fully in a series of studies relating to the availability of domestic gas, of car exhaust gas, and of guns. In all three cases, evidence is derived from time series studies and for two of them (guns and car exhaust gas) also from regional studies. Findings concerning displacement (substitution of one method for another) are reviewed and some pilot studies concerning

---

[4] An analogy here is provided by casino gambling in New Jersey. Casinos were permitted to open in Atlantic City only, recognizing the right of people to gamble if they wish to, but making them drive quite a distance to do so.

preferences for methods of suicide are presented. In the final chapter, a decision theory of suicide giving a greater role to the availability of lethal agents is outlined. A new model is also suggested for a public health approach to suicide prevention, the main plank of which is to make it more difficult for potential suicides to obtain the necessary lethal means.

2

Detoxification of Domestic Gas

As a result of the widespread replacement of coal gas by natural gas, public gas supplies in many countries are now free of toxic carbon monoxide. This detoxification of the gas supply constitutes a powerful natural experiment since poisoning by gas has been a frequently used method of suicide.

Nowhere have the results been more clearly demonstrated than in England and Wales. Until detoxification at the beginning of the 1960s, the suicide rate for men in England and Wales had been relatively steady during the century, though there was a peak in the Depression years and troughs during the two world wars. For women, the picture is one of a fairly steady increase in the suicide rate during the period, with smaller changes during the Depression and war years.

From 1963, as is shown in more detail later, the rate of suicide for both men and women declined markedly until the mid-1970s. Only Scotland and Greece, among 18 European countries studied by Sainsbury et al. (1980), showed similar though less pronounced declines. Since the mid-1970s, the female suicide rate has further declined, whereas the rate for males has risen, though not yet to the level of the early 1960s (Low et al., 1981).

Detoxification of domestic gas has considerably changed the distribution of different methods of suicide in England and Wales. For example, in 1960, suicides by domestic gas accounted for, respectively, just under and just over half of all male and female suicides. By 1980, only 0.2 percent of all suicides were by this method.[1]

---

[1] The most frequently used methods of suicide in 1980 for men were hanging, strangulation, and suffocation (accounting for nearly a third of the deaths), followed by poisoning with solid and liquid substances (accounting for nearly one-quarter of the deaths). Poisoning by gases other than ones in domestic use (mainly car exhaust fumes) accounted for roughly a further 15 percent of the male suicides. Women rarely used car exhaust gases (less than 3 percent of female suicides in 1980 were by this method) and used hanging and suffocation only about half as often as men. The most common method of suicide for women in 1980 (54 percent of the deaths) was poisoning by solid or liquid substances, most of which were pain killers, barbiturates, tranquillizers, and antidepressants. In contrast to the situation in the

(Footnote continued on next page)

Detoxification in England and Wales
Study 1

Following nationalization of the British gas industry in 1949, an extensive program of modernization was begun. More than 600 of the old and inefficient local gas works were closed, and many of the larger works were extended and linked together by a new system of mains (Williams, 1981). A program of research was also initiated to find more economical ways of producing gas which, at that time, was derived mainly from high-quality and increasingly scarce coal. Coal-based gas contained high concentrations of toxic carbon monoxide, but it was the search for economy that resulted in detoxification, the first stage of which began in the early 1950s.

At that time, less toxic gases (particularly oil-based gas), the fruits of the new production processes, began to be mixed with the existing gas. The average carbon monoxide content of the public gas supply gradually declined, with minor fluctuations, from a high of about 13 percent in the late 1950s to about 4 percent in 1968 (see Figure 2.1), which is when the second major change began to take effect.

This second change was the replacement of manufactured "town" gas by the then recently discovered natural gas from the North Sea. Natural gas consists largely of methane and is nonpoisonous. Because its combustion properties are different from those of manufactured gas, the two cannot be mixed, and natural gas had to be introduced area by area as each consumer's appliances were converted to burn natural gas. This massive conversion program, involving some 13.5 million consumers and 35 million appliances (Elliott, 1980), took nine years to complete.

While these changes were not motivated by considerations of safety, the side benefits of reduced toxicity were not wholly unanticipated. For example, an official government report (Morton, 1970) on the increased risks of undetected leaks and explosions associated with the use of natural gas nonetheless commented favorably on the greatly reduced likelihood of accidental poisonings, though suicide was not mentioned. The greater concern with accidents than with suicides is ironic because the latter outnumbered the former by more than three to one (Registrar General, 1961). Moreover, some "accidents" were probably suicides, and some explosions were undoubtedly the result of suicide attempts.[2]

(Footnote continued from previous page)

United States, where suicides with a gun account for about 55 percent of the total (Lester, 1984), firearms are rarely used in England and Wales. About 8 percent of male suicides and 0.4 percent of female suicides in England and Wales use guns (Bulusu and Alderson, 1984).

[2] One evening in 1970, one of us was disturbed at home by an explosion that destroyed the roof of a nearby apartment building. This turned out to be the result of escaped gas from a suicide attempt.

The gas industry's attitude seemed to reflect a general presumption: if people want to kill themselves, they will always find a way even if gas was not available. Therefore, the authorities could hardly be held responsible for people's intentional deaths as they might be for accidents. As we are trying to show in this volume, this presumption is ill-founded, though the gas authorities can hardly be criticized for being no wiser than anybody else at the time, including most experts on suicide.

Statistics

Table 2.1 shows the numbers of suicides by gas and by other methods in England and Wales from 1958 to 1977, whereas Figure 2.1 illustrates the relationship between the number of gas suicides and the annual average proportion of carbon monoxide in the domestic gas supply.

It can be seen that the decline in suicides by gas closely matches the reduced levels of toxicity. These suicides, which peaked in 1958 (2637) when the average carbon monoxide concentration was about 13 percent, declined to 23 in 1975 when the average carbon monoxide concentration was less than 1 percent. Overall levels of suicide did not decline until 1963 because the reduction in suicides by gas before then was masked by a general rise in other forms of suicide.

Though not perfect, the fit between toxicity and suicide could hardly have

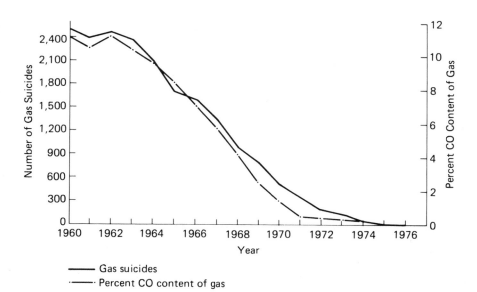

Figure 2.1. Gas Suicides in England and Wales, 1960–1976, and % CO content of domestic gas.

Table 2.1. Suicide by domestic gas, England and Wales, 1958–1977.

	All suicides	Suicides by domestic gas	
		Number	Percent
1958	5298	2637	49.8
1959	5207	2594	49.8
1960	5112	2499	48.9
1961	5200	2379	45.8
1962	5588	2469	44.2
1963	5714	2368	41.4
1964	5566	2088	37.5
1965	5161	1702	33.0
1966	4994	1593	31.9
1967	4711	1336	28.4
1968	4584	988	21.6
1969	4326	790	18.3
1970	3940	511	13.0
1971	3945	346	8.8
1972	3770	197	5.2
1973	3823	143	3.7
1974	3899	50	1.3
1975	3693	23	0.6
1976	3816	14	0.4
1977	3944	8	0.2

Source: Office of Population Censuses and Surveys, *Mortality Statistics, England Wales: Causes. Series DH2.* London: Her Majesty's Stationery Office, annual.

been any closer. In the first place, the figures for carbon monoxide concentrations are estimates for the United Kingdom as a whole, whereas conversion to natural gas took place later in Scotland, making the toxicity levels in England and Wales in later years somewhat lower than those suggested by the graph in Figure 2.1. Second, the measure of toxicity used is a relatively crude index of the availability of lethal gas because there were small daily and larger regional fluctuations in the actual toxicity of gas delivered to the homes, depending on the contribution to the public supply of different production centers.

Third, the measure of the average carbon monoxide concentration means somewhat different things before and after 1968, when conversion to natural gas began. Before 1968, the measure reflects the average toxicity of the gas in all homes. After 1968, an increasing proportion of homes (those that had been converted) had no carbon monoxide in their gas supply. Levels of carbon monoxide in unconverted homes would, therefore, have been higher than those suggested by the graph in Figure 2.1.

Fourth, certainty of death depends not just on the toxicity of the gas delivered, but also on the rate at which it is absorbed into the bloodstream (Drinker, 1938). This, in turn, depends on a range of other factors, including the size of the room, efforts to exclude fresh air, the amount of gas being released, and possibly the kind of appliance used. (Suicide may be easier with gas fires and ovens.) Since the number of these appliances decreased during the period in question (because of the widespread adoption of central heating and a general shift from gas to electric cooking), this might have led to fewer suicides in later years (see Study 2).

Although detoxification of the gas supply no doubt caused the decline in gas suicides, the more important and interesting question that we now pursue concerns the effect of detoxification on the suicide rate as a whole. Because of the powerful relationships with age and sex, data relating to suicide are presented for three age groups (younger than 24, 25 to 44, and 45 years and older) and separately for men (Figure 2.2) and women (Figure 2.3). In each case, rates are expressed per million of the population in the various age groups. The upper line for each age group represents suicides by all methods combined, domestic gas included; the lower line represents all suicides except those by domestic gas.

A number of conclusions can be drawn from inspection of these graphs:

1. The overall decline in male suicides between the early 1960s and the early 1970s is accounted for largely by the halving of suicides by the oldest age group because of the elimination of gas suicides. There is no evidence that, as gas suicides declined for this age group, other suicides increased.
2. The decline in gas suicides for the two younger groups of males during the same 10-year period is matched by increases in other kinds of suicide. However, these other suicides had been increasing before detoxification, which means that displacement from gas to other methods cannot wholly account for the observed pattern.
3. After 1975, when detoxification was all but complete, suicide rates for all three age groups of men show distinct increases.
4. For women, the decline in suicides by gas is not matched by increases in other kinds of suicide for the two older age groups, though it is for those under 24 years of age.
5. Unlike for men, rates of suicide for women have shown very little increase since 1975.

These facts indicate that, following detoxification, little displacement to other methods of suicide occurred, especially by women and older men, and thousands of lives were saved (6700, according to the calculations made by Wells [1981]). Nonetheless, some qualifications to both conclusions should be noted.

Concerning displacement, one possibility is that some undetected displacement occurred in the form of unsuccessful attempts using less lethal methods such as drug overdoses. This would be difficult to test because records of attempted suicide are incomplete and attempts appear to outnumber complete suicides to so great a degree (by an estimated 20 to one [Wells, 1981]), that, if all the latter were snatched from the jaws of death, the resulting increase in recorded attempts would be barely detectable (Kreitman, 1976).

Moreover, it is widely believed that most attempts constitute a distinct

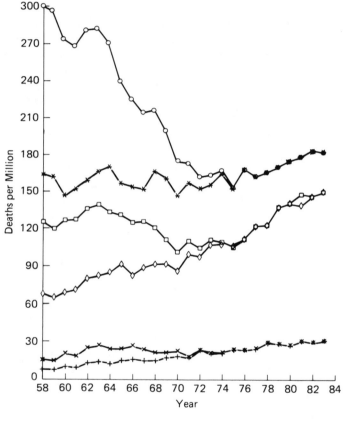

Figure 2.2. Suicides in England and Wales, 1958–1983.
Males: All methods and all methods minus domestic gas.

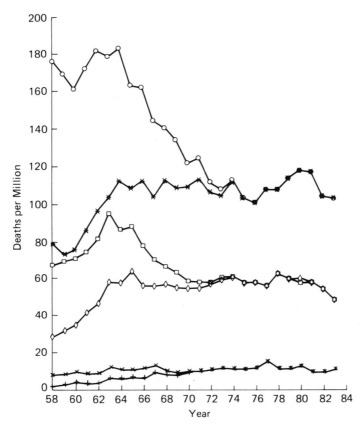

× <24 All
+ <24 All less gas
□ 25-44 All
◊ 25-44 All less gas
○ >45 All
∗ >45 All less gas

Figure 2.3. Suicides in England and Wales, 1958–1983.
Females: All methods and all methods minus domestic gas.

behavioral syndrome—"parasuicide" (Kreitman et al., 1969)—motivated less by a wish to die than by desire to obtain help with personal problems. The increases in "attempts" that appear to have taken place in recent decades, especially among young people and women (Weissman, 1974), therefore cannot be taken as evidence of displacement from gas unless—and this is a tragic possibility—some of those who died from gas were actually parasuicides who failed to realize its lethal nature. If this is so, as seems likely, detoxification achieved some of its effect by preventing such "accidental" deaths.[3]

Another possible source of undetected displacement relates in particular to elderly suicides. Some of these may have poisoned themselves (e.g., with barbiturates) when gas became unavailable; since poisonings among the elderly are more easily confused with natural deaths than are gasings (Patel, 1973), this may have artificially depressed the suicide statistics. However, concealment of such "displaced" poisoning will not be complete, and if the one method were readily substituted for the other, an inverse relation between the number of older suicides using gas and those using poisons might be expected. Richard Farmer (personal communication, 1986) checked this possibility using data reported in Low et al. (1981), but he found no significant relation.

On the saving of lives, some of the apparent gain might have been eliminated through "delayed" displacement; that is people prevented from using gas may commit suicide some years later. A disproportionate increase in suicides of older people throughout the 1980s is consistent with, though not necessarily proof of, this. It is too early yet to observe any full effect of delayed displacement, though to date the greatest increases have been among younger rather than older age groups. Furthermore, one cannot assume that the saving of lives achieved through detoxifications will continue. The suicidal population may identify new ways of killing themselves that share some of the advantages of gas. Indeed, there may already be some evidence of this in the increasing use of car exhaust fumes in England and Wales. For example, there were almost three times as many male suicides by this method in 1980 as in 1970 (Bulusu and Alderson, 1984).

Alternative Explanations for the Decline in Suicide

Detoxification was identified as the likely cause of the reduced suicide rate in one city in England, Birmingham, as long ago as 1972 (Hassall and

---

[3] An interesting case of someone who may have accidentally died making a suicide gesture with domestic gas is Sylvia Plath, an American poet, who died at the age of 30 in 1963 in London. She had left her husband, the British poet Ted Hughes, after finding out that he was having an affair. She took her two children to London and suffered through a cold and lonely winter. The plumbing froze, the children and she were sick, her poems were being rejected and her novel, *The Bell Jar*, which describes an earlier attempt at suicide when she was 20, was receiving only lukewarm reviews. Early one February morning she took milk and bread up to the children's rooms and went back to the kitchen where she sealed the door and put her head in the gas oven. Her physician had arranged for a nurse to visit her that morning, but the nurse did not break in with the assistance of workmen until late in the morning by which time Sylvia Plath was dead (Butscher, 1976). Alvarez, her friend and later a writer on suicide, believes that she had meant to survive, just as she had 10 years earlier, expecting the nurse to break in as soon as she arrived rather than delaying for a couple of hours (Alvarez, 1971). Had all of this occurred 10 years later, by which time domestic gas was being detoxified, Sylvia Plath might well have lived.

Trethowan, 1972). This was soon followed by the suggestion that reduced toxicity levels might account for the national decline in suicides (Malleson, 1973) and a little later by two detailed studies (Adelstein and Mardon, 1975; Kreitman, 1976) that reached this conclusion. Similar declines in overall levels of suicide had also been observed following detoxification of gas in Brisbane (Whitlock, 1975) and in Vienna where the overall rate declined about 30 percent (Farberow and Simon, 1969). In Vienna, the carbon monoxide content had been progressively reduced from 9.2 percent in 1965 to 6.8 percent in 1966 to between 4.5 and 2.5 percent in 1967. The effect on suicide is shown in the following statistics of suicides for Vienna as a whole:

	All suicides	Domestic gas suicides	
		Number	Percent
1961	347	199	57.3
1962	321	181	56.4
1963	308	202	65.6
1964	288	194	67.4
1965	349	175	50.1
1966	264	130	49.2
1967	246	80	32.5

Nevertheless, students of suicide have been reluctant to accept the detoxification hypothesis, many of whom have apparently been influenced by Stengel (1964), who observed, though without presenting data, that the transient decline in suicides following detoxification of gas in Basle was soon followed by a compensatory increase in drownings. Because such displacement has been seen as inevitable, explanations other than detoxification have been sought for the decline in the British suicide rate.

The first such explanation was that the decline in suicides may have been a result of a revision of the International Classification of Diseases (ICD) under which suicides are recorded (World Health Organization, 1967). The 1968 revision introduced a new category of "undetermined" cause of death, which could accommodate some of the marginal cases previously allocated to suicide. However, Kreitman (1976), Sainsbury (1983), and Bulusu and Alderson (1984) have concluded that, although a significant number of cases that previously would have been recorded as accidental poisonings began to be placed in the new "undetermined" category, the ICD revision seems to have had little effect on the recording of suicide. For example, Kreitman found that the decrement in suicides between 1967 and 1968 was no greater than that between any other years in the period 1960 to 1971 for all but 2 of 14 sex–age subgroups. This result was repeated when carbon monoxide suicides were examined alone.

A second hypothesis was that improvements in resuscitation and treatment of poisoning, together with the establishment of more efficient ambulance services after World War II, resulted in saving the lives of some potential suicides. Though not an implausible idea, no supporting controlled study could be found by Brown (1979). Moreover, these improvements would be more likely to have achieved a reduction in suicides using less lethal methods (such as overdosing) than in those using gas, most of whom are discovered already dead.

Brown (1979) also investigated a third idea, that the improved treatment of suicidal patients—for example, through the wider use of antidepressants in both general practice and the aftercare of mental hospital patients—may have brought about the drop in completed suicides (see also Barraclough, 1972). Again, he was unable to find any supporting evidence, but Fox (1975) has pointed out that an unintended consequence of the wider prescribing of antidepressants is to supply more people with the means of killing themselves.

A fourth explanation was that the declining suicide rates reflected the rapid development of the Samaritans, an organization providing a lay crisis intervention service for depressed and suicidal people. As mentioned in Chapter 1, Bagley (1968) found that 15 towns with branches of the Samaritans had experienced a fall in their average suicide rates, while suicides in a set of comparison towns had risen. Brown (1979) pointed out that this study might show only that some third factor, such as social cohesiveness, could both increase the likelihood of the formation of a Samaritans branch and reduce the incidence of suicide in the same town. Nonetheless, Bagley's study was eagerly seized on by the Samaritans and their supporters (e.g., Fox, 1975); it was called into serious question only nine years later by a replication study published by Barraclough, Jennings, and Moss (1977). Using a much larger sample of both Samaritans towns and controls and three different methods of matching, the new study could find no evidence of any preventive effect. Another major difficulty for the Samaritans hypothesis is that the decline in the suicide trend began to level off in 1971 while the numbers of Samaritans branches and their clients continued to increase until at least 1975 (Brown, 1979).

A fifth hypothesis, that the suicide decline was due to improved social and economic conditions in Britain (Sainsbury, Jenkins, and Levey, 1980), might appear somewhat perverse in that the Britain of the late 1960s and early 1970s is commonly thought to have been marked by "industrial unrest, rising unemployment and a constant state of economic crisis" (Fox, 1975, p. 9). Indeed, it is clear that the 35 percent drop in the suicide rate between 1963 and 1975 occurred despite a 50 percent increase in the unemployment rate during the same period (Boor, 1981; Kreitman and Platt, 1984). Moreover, one other important social indicator, the rate of recorded crime, suggested a markedly deteriorating situation with a 60 percent increase between 1965 and 1974.

The starting point of Sainsbury and associates' study, however, was the observation that only Greece, among 18 European countries, had experienced a similar decline in suicide. Using a discriminant function analysis, they found that changes in the suicide rates in European countries between the periods 1961–63 and 1972–74 were correlated with socioeconomic changes, as measured by such variables as the proportion of young people and working women in the population, the ownership of television receivers, rates of unemployment, divorce, and illegitimacy. Leaving aside whether suicide figures can be reliably used for international comparisons (in relation to Sainsbury's research, see Farmer and Rohde [1980]), the study is open to numerous technical criticisms. These concern the selection of socioeconomic variables and the rationale of their relation to suicide, the questionable division of countries into those with "high increases" in suicide and others with "low increases or decreases" for purposes of the discriminant function analysis, and the use of this analysis with 15 variables but only 18 cases. At best, the study demonstrates that socioeconomic change may be responsible for some changes in suicide rates. However, it does not provide an alternative explanation for the decline in the British suicide rate during the period in question: based on the analysis presented, the suicide rates of England and Wales should have increased more than those of seven other countries, but in reality they showed the greatest decrease of all.

Besides these alternative explanations for the decline in suicide, some evidence apparently inconsistent with the gas detoxification hypothesis has also been produced. In the first place, it has been shown that detoxification of the gas supply in the Netherlands did not produce a drop in the overall level of suicide in that country. On the face of it, this calls into question the generality of the detoxification effect, but Study 2, reported later, shows that the lack of apparent effect on the overall rates of suicide could have been the result of a general rise in suicidal motivation in the Netherlands. Second, Sainsbury (1986) has claimed that towns in England and Wales whose gas supplies were not detoxified until relatively late showed the same patterns of suicide as those whose supplies were detoxified earlier. However, Sainsbury's claim does not appear to be well supported by the data. Only 12 towns (all of which had roughly the same levels of carbon monoxide in their gas supplies in 1958, but five of which had lower levels by 1967) were included in the study, and between them these accounted for only a small number of suicides (135 in 1958 and 142 in 1967). Moreover, the study relates to a period before the conversion to natural gas, and the "detoxified" towns still had a small percentage (about 5 percent) of carbon monoxide in their (manufactured) gas supplies. This level of carbon monoxide is sufficient to kill, even though death may take longer. Unfortunately, no data are presented about the number of suicides resulting from domestic gas in either group of towns.

Summary

In sum, it is clear that substantial reductions in the carbon monoxide content of the public gas supply in Britain led to the virtual disappearance of suicide by domestic gas. Because few of the people stopped from using gas found another way of killing themselves, a substantial decline (approaching 40 percent) in the overall number of suicides resulted. The various alternative hypotheses to explain the decline and some supposedly contradictory facts are not well-supported by available evidence.

Since the mid-1970s, suicides have gradually increased and, for men, have now surpassed the levels existing before detoxification of the gas supply. In light of the evidence concerning a general rise in suicidal behavior, and also because of the increased use of some more novel means of suicide (such as car exhaust gases), it is not unreasonable to think that present levels of suicide would have been much greater without detoxification.

Detoxification in Scotland and the Netherlands
Study 2

Although detoxification of the gas supply clearly led to a substantial decline of suicide in England and Wales, the generality of the detoxification effect has been called into question by the experience of some other countries. Reductions in *domestic gas* suicide have invariably been observed, but *overall* rates of suicide have not always declined. For example, while overall rates of suicide did decline following detoxification in Australia (Whitlock, 1975) and Vienna (Farberow and Simon, 1969), they did not in the Netherlands (World Health Organization, 1982) and may not have done in Basle (as claimed by Stengel, 1964). More particularly, detoxification had less effect on the overall rate of suicide in Scotland than in the remainder of Great Britain (Kreitman, 1976).

These facts do not, of course, invalidate the findings for England and Wales. It is quite possible that the removal of a particular method of suicide in one country might have a different effect from that of its removal in another. Thus, it could be argued that detoxification might have had a larger effect on the overall suicide statistics in England and Wales than elsewhere (1) because of the stronger link in that culture between the idea of suicide and "putting one's head in the gas oven," and (2) because a nation widely regarded as conservative in its way of life would also be conservative in its chosen ways of death.

These possibilities may account for the lack of displacement in England and Wales, but its absence has generally been thought to be a result of the particular advantages of domestic gas as a method of suicide. Gas was widely available, required little preparation or courage, did not disfigure, and was painless and bloodless (Brown, 1979). These advantages are likely to appeal generally to the suicidally inclined, and one might, therefore, expect limited displacement in any culture following detoxification.

For these reasons, the present study investigated an alternative hypothesis to that of displacement for the apparently more limited effect of detoxification in some countries: that the effect of the drop in gas suicides on the overall suicide rate was masked not by displacement, but by an unrelated general rise in other forms of suicide. For purely arithmetic reasons, such masking is most likely to have occurred where suicide by gas initially formed a smaller proportion of the total—as, for example, in the Netherlands.

This hypothesis was examined in the context of a comparison of the patterns of suicide for England and Wales, Scotland, and the Netherlands during 1960 through 1975, years encompassing the different periods of detoxification in the three countries. Detoxification had its main effect on carbon monoxide levels as follows:

England and Wales: between 1962 and 1971 (a decline from 11.5 to 0.5 percent);
Scotland: between 1962 and 1975 (from 13.2 to 0.7 percent);
Netherlands: between 1963 and 1968 (from 12.3 to 0.2 percent).

In the light of criticisms frequently made about international comparisons of suicide rates (Farmer and Rohde, 1980), as well as of the controversy surrounding differences in the suicide rates of Scotland and of England and Wales (Ross and Kreitman, 1975), it should be noted that the present study compares patterns of change *within* each country consequent to detoxification rather than rates of suicide *between* countries. Such a comparison should be less vulnerable to variations between countries in the procedures for certifying and recording suicide. More problematic for this study may be the accuracy of figures concerning the toxicity of gas supplies in each country, since some of these had to be estimated.[4]

Effect on Gas Suicides

It can be seen from Table 2.2 and Figure 2.4 that, in all three countries, detoxification of the gas supply resulted in the virtual elimination of suicide by gas. There is a remarkably close fit between the decline in the carbon monoxide content of the total gas supply and the decline in the number of gas suicides (for England and Wales $r = 0.99$; for Scotland, $r = 0.94$; and for Netherlands, $r = 0.97$). Two alternative measures of toxicity, based on the yearly proportion of homes in each country supplied with manufactured gas and the average carbon monoxide content of gas supplied to just those homes, produced a slightly poorer but still close fit with the number of suicides by gas.

---

[4] All data sources are described in Clarke and Mayhew (1989).

Table 2.2. Suicides and carbon monoxide content of domestic gas: England and Wales, Scotland, and the Netherlands, 1960–1975.

	England and Wales			Scotland			The Netherlands		
Year	All suicides	Domestic gas suicides	CO content of gas[a]	All suicides	Domestic gas suicides	CO content of gas[a]	All suicides	Domestic gas suicides	CO content of gas[b]
1960	5112	2499	11.3	408	200	11.1	762	187	12.5
1961	5200	2379	10.6	409	199	12.4	774	176	12.5
1962	5588	2469	11.5	473	219	13.1	781	167	12.5
1963	5714	2368	11.7	445	149	11.0	742	129	12.3
1964	5566	2088	9.8	425	119	8.6	792	141	11.3
1965	5161	1702	8.6	415	139	9.0	850	114	8.2
1966	4994	1593	7.2	413	118	7.5	881	68	4.0
1967	4711	1336	5.8	391	87	6.7	783	27	1.0
1968	4584	988	4.2	373	59	7.0	806	12	0.2
1969	4326	790	2.5	362	53	7.2	942	8	0.1
1970	3940	511	1.4	397	71	5.9	1051	5	0
1971	3945	346	0.5	378	55	3.4	1090	6	0
1972	3770	197	0.4	421	37	1.5	1094	10	0
1973	3823	143	0.3	436	21	1.2	1164	5	0
1974	3899	50	0.2	437	21	1.0	1247	9	0
1975	3693	23	0.0	427	11	0.7	1219	11	0

[a] Unpublished estimates by British Gas. These figures were calculated by weighting the proportions of different kinds of gas supplied in each year by the following estimated values for CO content: natural gas and refinery gas—0%; coal gas—7.5%; blue water gas—40%; carburetted water gas—30%; oil gasification (cyclic)—20%; oil gasification (continuous)—4%; producer gas, etc.—23%; coke oven gas—7%.
[b] Calculated on the basis of the following data supplied by Veg-Gasinstituut for proportions of connections receiving natural gas and an average CO content for manufactured gas of 14%: 1961—10.0%; 1962—10.4%; 1963—11.6%; 1964—19.3%; 1965—42.7%; 1966—72.8%; 1967—93.6%; 1968—99.1%; 1969—99.3%.

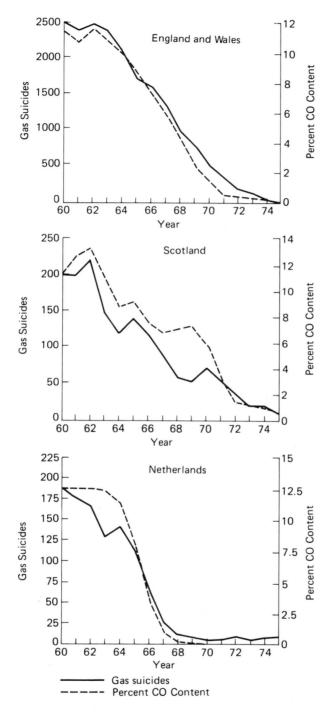

Figure 2.4. Gas suicides and CO content of gas, 1960–1975.

Effect on Overall Rates of Suicide

Figure 2.5 presents crude suicide rates per million of the population in each country for all methods of suicide (top line in each graph) and for all methods minus domestic gas.

For England and Wales, it can be seen that the overall rate of suicide fell by 38 percent between 1963 and 1975 (from 121 to 75 per million). During the same period, a small 5 percent rise occurred in suicide rates by all methods other than domestic gas. If this rise represents displacement to other methods for suicide, clearly this involves only very few of the potential suicides.

For Scotland, the maximum decline in the overall suicide rate was between 1962 and 1971 when it declined by about 30 percent (from 91 to 72 per million). Thereafter, the overall suicide rate began to rise again and had reached 93 percent of its 1962 level by 1975. Thus, the decline in the overall suicide rate in Scotland was smaller and of shorter duration than the decline in England and Wales.

These changes are consistent with the hypothesis that the rise in the overall suicide rate in Scotland after 1972 was the result of a general increase in the tendency to suicide during the period under study. Evidence for this is the fact that the suicide rate by all methods except domestic gas doubled in Scotland between 1960 and 1975, from 40 to 80 per million. The effect of this increase on the overall suicide rate between 1962 and 1971 would have been masked by the decline in suicides resulting from detoxification of domestic gas.

For the Netherlands, the period of detoxification, 1963 to 1968, was accompanied by almost no change in the overall suicide rate (from 61 to 62 per million) despite the elimination of domestic gas suicides. During the same period, nongas suicides increased by about 30 percent, which could be interpreted as evidence of displacement from domestic gas. However, these suicides also increased at about the same rate *after* detoxification, from 61 per million in 1968 to 88 per million in 1975. Once again, therefore, these facts are consistent with the hypothesis that a general increase in the tendency to complete suicide in the Netherlands during the period of detoxification masked the effect of detoxification on the overall rate of suicide.

Change in Methods

Closer analysis of the methods employed in suicide might, in theory, clarify the reasons for the smaller effect of detoxification on the overall rate of suicide in Scotland and the apparent absence of an effect in the Netherlands. For example, if it were found that the decrease in domestic gas poisoning had been matched by an increase in a similar method, such as poisonings by solid or liquid substances, this might be taken as evidence of displacement.

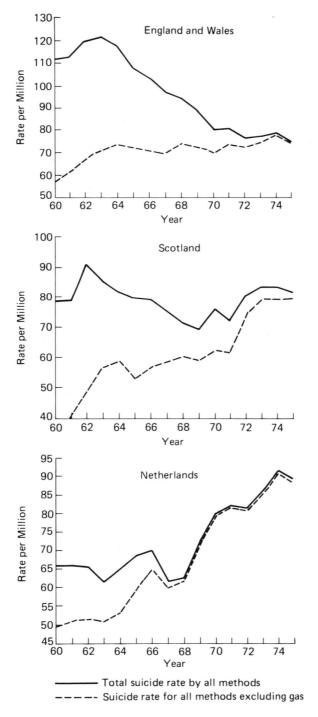

Figure 2.5. Suicide rates by method, 1960–1975.

On the other hand, if there were a more general rise in all forms of suicide, or in forms such as jumping from high buildings that are rather different from domestic gas poisoning, then this might be seen as evidence of a coincident rather than a consequent rise in these suicides.

Unfortunately, the analysis do not support either explanation unequivocally. In the Netherlands during the period, there was a substantial increase in poisoning by solid and liquid substances (from 71 in 1960 to 295 in 1975), but about half of this increase occurred in the period *after* detoxification. There was also a substantial rise (from 18 in 1960 to 95 in 1975) in jumping from high buildings and a general increase in all other forms of suicide.

In Scotland, consistent with a displacement hypothesis, most of the increase in forms of suicide other than domestic gas poisonings was accounted for by an increase in poisonings by solid and liquid substances (which increased from 51 in 1960 to 200 in 1975). Inconsistent with displacement, however, is the fact that half of this increase had already occurred by 1962, before the start of detoxification.

Gas Suicide in the Netherlands Prior to Detoxification

Cultural traditions may have meant that domestic gas poisoning played less of a part in Dutch suicide, but there may also have been less opportunity to use gas, a supposition supported by the fact that accidental deaths by domestic gas poisoning were also markedly lower in the Netherlands. From 1955 to 1959 these deaths averaged about 5.4 per million of the population, compared with an average of 18.3 per million for England and Wales and 20 per million for Scotland. Although the gas supply in the Netherlands was no less toxic in 1960, fewer Dutch households received a toxic gas supply—about 59 percent compared with about 75 percent in England and Wales and 66 percent in Scotland (Clarke and Mayhew, 1989). In addition, fewer Dutch homes in the early 1960s appear to have had gas cookers or gas fires, the favorite appliances for use in suicide. Approximately 4 percent of Dutch homes had gas fires in the early 1960s (Peebles, 1980), compared with about 12 percent in England and Wales and 10 percent in Scotland. (These latter figures derive from data for the conversion program [Elliott, 1980].)

As for cookers, about 90 percent of homes supplied by gas in England and Wales and 80 percent in Scotland had a gas cooker in 1964 (Elliott, 1980), whereas the estimated figure provided by the Dutch Veg-Gasinstituut for the Netherlands is about 50 percent (J. A. Vernout, personal communication).

Important design differences also made Dutch appliances more difficult to use for suicide. Gas cookers in the Netherlands were more likely to have downward-opening doors, which makes suicide more difficult, whereas cookers in Great Britain were more likely to have side-opening doors. And, unlike most British gas fires, which had an open flame, the flame of Dutch gas fires was enclosed behind a fixed glass door; again, this would have made suicide more difficult (J. A. Vernout, personal communication).

Detoxification in the United States
Study 3

Given the attention devoted to the topic in other countries, it is surprising that the effects of detoxification seem not to have been studied previously in the United States. We therefore decided to examine the results of the gradual switch to natural gas that began in the United States some 30 years before its occurrence in England and Wales.

Unfortunately, because of revisions made in the classifications of deaths used in the *Vital Statistics*, it was not possible to go back earlier than 1946 when, according to the *Statistical Abstracts of the United States*, just over 45 percent of all gas customers were already using nontoxic natural gas. By 1970, nearly 99 percent of all customers were supplied by natural gas.

Our examination of the figures for the period 1946–1970 quickly revealed two facts (Table 2.3). First, the rates of suicide by domestic gas decreased as more customers were switched to natural gas ($r = -0.87$), and these suicides were virtually eliminated by the end of the period. Second, the rate of suicides by motor vehicle exhaust gases greatly increased over the same period ($r = 0.92$). Indeed, on the face of it, there appeared to have been a straight switch between the two methods, with the rate of motor vehicle exhaust suicides increasing as that for domestic gas suicides declined ($r = -0.94$). Given that the sum of the two suicide rates during the period did not change a great deal (from 1.273 to 1.025 per 100,000, or a decline of about 19 percent), displacement between the two methods appears to have been considerable.

Before reaching the conclusion that displacement did occur, however, one further possibility must be considered—that the increase in car exhaust suicides might have occurred *independent* of any decline in suicide by domestic gas. The reason for this is the great increase in car ownership that took place following World War II. (We show in Chapter 3 that the use of car exhaust gas to commit suicide is strongly related to car ownership.) Cars per capita of the population increased steadily during the period ($r = 0.99$), from 0.210 in 1946 to 0.435 in 1970 (See Table 2.3).

According to this alternative hypothesis, therefore the decline in domestic gas suicides and the increase in car exhaust suicides were independent phenomena, resulting from two separate processes—the decline of toxic domestic gas, on the one hand, and the increase in car ownership, on the other.

Some evidence supporting this alternative hypothesis is provided by examining sex differences. For men, in 1950 for example, the suicide rate with car exhaust was 1.092 and that with domestic gas was 0.854, giving a

Table 2.3. Suicide rates using domestic gas and motor vehicle exhaust and the extent of natural gas usage by consumers in the United States, 1964–1970.

	Cars per capita	Percentage of custom- ers using natural gas	Domestic gas	Motor vehicle exhaust	All gas	All other methods	Overall
			Suicide rates per 100,000 per year by				
1946	0.210	45.4%	0.926	0.347	1.273	10.208	11.481
1947	0.214	47.6%	0.834	0.341	1.175	10.303	11.478
1948	0.227	51.5%	0.811	0.426	1.237	9.909	11.146
1949	0.244	53.9%	0.749	0.490	1.239	10.142	11.381
1950	0.265	60.8%	0.727	0.604	1.331	9.929	11.260
1951	0.276	66.0%	0.481	0.695	1.176	9.096	10.272
1952	0.278	72.2%	0.330	0.612	0.942	8.938	9.880
1953	0.290	75.9%	0.239	0.747	0.986	8.969	9.955
1954	0.297	78.7%	0.225	0.791	1.016	9.017	10.033
1955	0.314	81.6%	0.190	0.745	0.935	9.166	10.101
1956	0.321	86.1%	0.153	0.797	0.950	8.953	9.903
1957	0.325	89.3%	0.199	0.771	0.890	8.781	9.671
1958	0.325	90.3%	0.118	0.890	1.008	9.581	10.589
1959	0.334	91.5%	0.093	0.909	1.002	9.476	10.478
1960	0.341	92.8%	0.103	0.910	1.013	9.526	10.539
1961	0.345	93.9%	0.096	0.977	1.073	9.270	10.343
1962	0.354	94.5%	0.095	0.994	1.089	9.744	10.833
1963	0.365	95.7%	0.092	1.105	1.197	9.807	11.004
1964	0.375	97.4%	0.044	1.070	1.114	9.615	10.729
1965	0.387	98.0%	0.080	1.091	1.171	9.898	11.069
1966	0.397	98.2%	0.079	1.041	1.120	9.707	10.827
1967	0.405	98.3%	0.074	1.031	1.105	9.627	10.732
1968	0.416	98.5%	0.023	0.953	0.976	9.672	10.648
1969	0.429	98.6%	0.030	1.007	1.037	9.997	11.034
1970	0.435	98.6%	0.021	1.025	1.046	10.405	11.451

total of 1.946. In 1960 these rates were, respectively, 1.547 and 0.134, giving a total of 1.681, a slight decrease from 1950 in the overall total, indicating that the decline in the use of domestic gas was largely, but not completely, offset by the increase in the use of car exhaust.

For women, however, the figures are very different. In 1950, the suicide rate for women using car exhaust was 0.125 and the rate with domestic gas was 0.607, giving a total of 0.732. In 1960, the rates were, respectively, 0.287 and 0.072, giving a total of 0.359. Thus, the total use of car exhaust and domestic gas by women declined tremendously through the 1950s. The decrease in the use of domestic gas was offset very little by an increase in the use of car exhaust.

This analysis of sex differences therefore shows that displacement cannot be the sole reason for the increase in car exhaust suicides. Further light on the extent of any displacement might be shed by comparing car exhaust suicides from different areas of the country in which the gas supply was or was not switched to natural gas after 1946. To the extent that displacement plays a part, the increase in car exhaust suicides in those areas where natural gas was introduced post-1946 should be greater than in the other areas. If the increases in car exhaust suicides are of the same order between the two areas, then displacement cannot provide the explanation.

This analysis, which is beyond our present resources, is clearly an important one to undertake. In the meanwhile, some important points need to be made. First, even if some displacement from domestic gas suicides to car exhaust suicides took place, it was not complete. Second, though it is tempting to concede that displacement between two such apparently similar methods is to be expected, the differences between the methods should not be overlooked. In particular, car exhaust suicide requires more technical knowledge (which may deter women) and many classes of people (for example, the poor or very old) do not have widespread access to cars. Third, the existence of displacement between the two methods in the United States would not invalidate conclusions concerning lack of displacement in Britain. One important difference, or course, is that in England and Wales gas suicide was well entrenched as the dominant method, with about half of all suicides using the method at one time. In the United States, only about 11 percent of suicides in 1946 used this method. In other words, there may be special reasons why displacement did not occur to any appreciable extent following detoxification in England and Wales. The more understanding we have of such matters, the more confidently we can predict the effect of restricting lethal agents and the more carefully we can pursue such preventive measures.

Conclusions

The research reported in this chapter has shown that the very substantial decline, approaching 40 percent, in the overall rate of suicide in England and Wales from 1963 to 1975 was the result of detoxification of the domestic gas supply. The research also suggests that the lesser effect of detoxification on the overall rate of suicide in Scotland and the Netherlands may have been the result not of displacement to other methods of suicide but of coincident increases in the tendency to commit suicide in those countries during the period of detoxification.

The decline in the United States in the availability of toxic domestic gas being accompanied by an increase in car ownership, as well as by a change in the pattern of suicide, may explain why detoxification of domestic gas does not always lead to a decrease in the overall suicide rate.

If, as the availability of one method for suicide decreases, the availability of another method increases, the overall rate of suicide may not change much. Furthermore, it is by no means clear to what extent *individuals* will switch methods for suicide. For example, there are no data to test whether those who eventually used car exhaust for suicide in the United States in the 1950s and 1960s might have used domestic gas had it remained toxic or whether they would have only used car exhaust as a method.

Furthermore, the choice of a method for suicide may not be affected simply by the number of people who possess the technology; it may also be affected by suggestion. For example, mountains and cliffs are (relatively) permanent objects. However, most people do not perceive them as available methods for suicide until publicity is given to someone who uses this particular venue for suicide. That venue is then perceived by others as an available method, and the site occasionally becomes a mecca for suicides.

Thus, not only must a method for suicide become more available—for example, more people owning cars—but people must also learn that car exhaust is a way of committing suicide. These issues are explored further in subsequent chapters.

3

The Toxicity of Car Exhaust

It was shown in the previous chapter that the increase of cars in the United States following World War II was accompanied by an increase in suicides by car exhausts. A further natural experiment relating to the availability of this method for suicide is provided by the introduction of exhaust emission controls in the United States. These controls were intended to reduce the level of air pollution by requiring new vehicles to be fitted with devices to remove, or greatly reduce, the toxic agents in exhaust gases, including hydrocarbons, nitrogen oxides, and carbon monoxide. It is the latter gas which is fatal in sufficiently high concentrations in a confined space, such as the passenger compartment of a car or a closed garage.

Emission controls were introduced by the federal government for all new cars in 1968, though some states particularly troubled by air pollution, such as California, had imposed them a few years earlier. The federal standards became progressively stricter so that the exhaust gases of newer cars were required to be much cleaner than those of cars produced in the early years of emission controls. Thus, the carbon monoxide content of the exhaust gas of 1984 cars had to be reduced to only 4 percent of that of pre-emission–control cars, whereas the corresponding figure for 1968 cars was 40 percent. Emission controls have made it more difficult to complete suicide with the newer cars, and as a consequence reports have appeared recently of failed suicide attempts using car exhaust (Landers, 1981; Hay and Bornstein, 1984).

The research reported in this chapter was designed to examine the overall effect of emission controls on this common method for suicide in the United States and to compare rates of car exhaust suicides in the United States with those in Britain (excluding Northern Ireland), where emission controls have yet to be introduced. We begin by examining the variation in suicides by car exhaust across the United States.

Car Exhaust Suicides in the United States
Study 4

In this study we explored the variation in the rate of suicide by car exhaust over the continental United States, to see whether this rate was related to the availability of cars.

The most likely correlate of the rate of suicide by car exhaust was the extent of car ownership, measured here as the number of cars per capita. Earlier writers, such as Drinker (1938), argued that the use of car exhaust for suicide was more common in rural areas because houses were more likely to have garages, and so we included the percentage of each state's population living in urban areas in the study. We also included the approximate latitude and longitude of each state in the data analysis since Lester (1983) has shown that suicide rates in the United States vary with both latitude and longitude.

We obtained the number of car exhaust suicides in each state of the United States in 1980 from data tapes provided by the National Center for Health Statistics (which puts the roughly 2 million death certificates each year on magnetic data tapes). We found the population of each state and the percentage of the population living in urban areas in reports from the U.S. Census Bureau (1984). We found the latitude and longitude of each state capital in a standard United States geographical atlas. The numbers of cars registered in each state for 1980 were obtained from a report of the Federal Highway Administration (1982).

The results are summarized in Table 3.1. The rate of suicide from car exhaust was related to the number of cars per capita in the states (Pearson $r = 0.36$; one-tailed $p < 0.01$) and to the percentage of the population living in urban areas ($r = 0.25$; $p < 0.05$). Rates of suicide from car exhaust were higher in the northern states ($r = 0.52$, $p < 0.001$) but showed no east–west variation ($r = 0.12$).

Table 3.1. Correlations between suicide rates and car ownership over the United States in 1980.

	Car exhaust suicide rate	Other suicide rate	Total suicide rate
Cars per capita	0.36[a]	0.04	0.13
Percentage urban population	0.25[a]	0.02	0.08
North–south	0.52[a]	−0.22	−0.09
East-west	0.12	0.57[a]	0.60[a]
Car exhaust suicide rate	—	−0.13	0.13
Other suicide rate	−0.13	—	0.97[a]
Total suicide rate	0.13	0.97[a]	—

[a] Statistically significant at the 5% level or better.

These correlations are very different from those for the total suicide rate and the suicide rate by methods other than car exhaust, which showed no association with the number of cars per capita or the percentage of the population living in urban areas. These rates showed an east–west variation and no north–south variation.

The study therefore showed that, in states with a smaller per capita ownership of cars, the suicide rate by car exhaust is lower; this suggests once again that the toxicity and availability of a method for suicide appears to be related to the frequency of its use for suicide. Where there are fewer cars, fewer people use car exhaust for suicide.

This topic is difficult to study in America because car ownership is so widespread. Almost every family has a car, sometimes more than one. Even in poorer regions of the country, backyards are often strewn with cars in various states of repair (or disrepair), which, incidentally, probably produce car exhaust with very high concentrations of carbon monoxide. It would be of interest, therefore, to repeat this study of variation in car exhaust suicides in a nation where car ownership was less common (with fewer people having access to a car), in countries where emission controls have not yet been imposed, and at earlier periods of time in America when car ownership was less common.

Comparison of the United States and Great Britain
Study 5

In this study, we used time series data to examine the overall effect of emission controls on the rates of car exhaust suicide in the United States and to compare rates with those in England, Wales, and Scotland, where emission controls have not yet been introduced. For both countries, we used the number of cars in use as the measure of opportunity for car exhaust suicide. For the United States, however, we calculated an "adjusted" measure of cars in use to take into account the progressive effect of emission controls in reducing the toxicity of the exhaust gases of the newer cars.

For the United States, we obtained the numbers of motor vehicle exhaust suicides for 1950 to 1984 from the annual volumes of the *Vital Statistics of the United States*. For Great Britain, the category for suicide by car exhaust is slightly broader: "suicides by poisoning with other gases." However, in 1979, 95 percent of suicides by this means involved car exhaust. We obtained suicide data for Scotland from the *Annual Report of the Registrar General for Scotland* (1950–1984) and for England and Wales from the *Statistical Review of England & Wales, Part 1B, Medical* (1950–1973) and the *Mortality Statistics, DH4* (1974–1984).

We obtained population figures for the United States from the *Statistical Abstract of the United States: 1986* and for Great Britain (midyear estimates) from volumes of the *Annual Abstract of Statistics*. We found the number of "cars and vans registered in private use" in Great Britain in the *Annual Abstract of Statistics*. For the United States, we found figures for "cars in operation" in *Facts and Figures*, the annual reports of the Motor Vehicle Manufacturers Association (MVMA).

The Adjusted Measure of Cars for the United States

The MVMA figures for "cars in operation" are listed by year of manufacture or, more strictly, by model year. This, together with the carbon monoxide emission standards holding for each year, permits calculation of an "adjusted" measure of cars in operation that takes into account the progressively reduced toxicity of car produced from 1968 onwards.

The emission standards, also listed in the MVMA annual reports, are as follows: 1968–1971 carbon monoxide content of exhaust gases in all new cars to be reduced to 40 percent of pre-emission–control levels (that is, before 1968); for 1972–1974 to 33 percent; for 1975–1979 to 18 percent; for 1980 to 8 percent; and for 1981–1984 to 4 percent.

The effect of applying these standards to cars in operation would, for example, mean that each 1981 car would contribute only 4 percent as much to the "adjusted" 1981 measure of cars in operation as each pre-emission–control car. To illustrate the procedure involved, the calculation for 1981 is shown here:

Model year	Cars in operation in 1981 (thousands)	Carbon monoxide standard	Adjusted measure of cars in operation (thousands)
1968	7,920	100%	7,920.00
1968–1971	15,171	40%	6,068.40
1972–1974	23,299	33%	7,688.67
1975–1979	45,491	18%	8,188.38
1980	8,818	8%	705.44
1981	5,140	4%	205.60
Total	105,839		30,776.49

It can be seen that the "adjusted" measure of cars in operation for 1981 was 30,776,490 compared with the actual number of cars in operation of about 105,839,000. In calculating adjusted measures, it was not possible to take into account the fact (mentioned earlier) that for a few years before emission standards were introduced nationwide in 1968 some states had introduced controls and some new models carried emission controls before they were required to.

Results and Discussion

Figure 3.1 shows that the rate of car exhaust suicide in the United States increased fairly steadily from about 6 per million of the population per year to about 11 per million in the mid-1960s. Thereafter, the rate gradually declined to about 9 per million in the 1980s. The rate for Great Britain was initially much lower than in the United States—less than one car exhaust suicide per million per year in 1950. Until 1970, the rate increased gradually to about three per million. Thereafter it increased much more rapidly, surpassing the rate in the United States in the later 1970s to nearly 17 per million in 1984.

The picture revealed by Figure 3.1 is essentially consistent with the idea that emission controls in the United States have reduced the opportunity for suicide by car exhaust gas. The fact that the decline in these suicides began slightly before nationwide controls were introduced probably reflects the earlier introduction of emission controls in some states and on some new cars. However, Figure 3.1 also raises some questions. In particular, why did the rate of car exhaust suicides increase in the United States until the beginning of emission controls? And why did the similar steady increase in these suicides in Britain until the beginning of the 1970s greatly escalate thereafter?

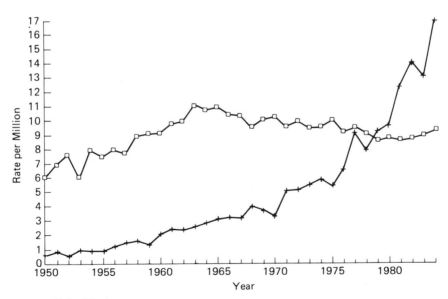

□ United States
+ Great Britain

Figure 3.1. Rates of car exhaust suicide, United States and Great Britain, 1950–1984.

Some light is shed on the first question in Figure 3.2, which shows car exhaust suicides in the United States for 1950 to 1984 in relation to cars in operation and the "adjusted" measure of cars in operation. (Number of car exhaust suicides are standardized against a population base for 1950.) As expected, the increase in the number of car exhaust suicides matches closely the increase in the number of cars in operation until the advent of emission controls in the mid-1960s. The fact that the subsequent decline in exhaust suicides does not as closely fit the decline in opportunities, as measured by the "adjusted" number of cars in operation, is more difficult to explain.

One reason may be that between 1965 and 1984 the overall motivation to commit suicide increased, as is suggested by the rise in the rate of suicide from 9.8 per 100,000 per year to 12.4. This may have increased the number of people trying to kill themselves with car exhaust gases.

Possibly more important, the "adjusted" measure of cars in operation might exaggerate the reduction in opportunities for car exhaust suicides. After all, potential suicides could either disconnect the emission controls or inhale exhaust fumes for much longer periods. Moreover, in a nation of two-car families, many people who own a new car may also have access to a toxic pre-emission–control car. If we consider a family with two cars, one from 1979 and one from 1981, the toxicity of their cars is not (18 + 4 percent) divided by 2 = 11 percent. It is 18 percent, the toxicity of the more toxic car. Thus, suicidal deaths from car exhaust can be expected to decline

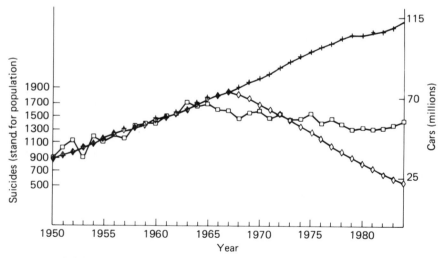

Figure 3.2. Exhaust suicides and cars in operation, United States, 1950–1984.

more dramatically only when the number of older toxic cars in use drops substantially.

Some support for this line of reasoning can be found by examining the relationship between numbers of cars and accidental poisoning deaths from car exhaust. The number of such deaths should correlate more closely with the "adjusted" measure of cars in operation since, in these cases, the victims would not have sought out the more toxic cars or found ways around the emission controls. The *Vital Statistics* shows that accidental deaths involving poisoning by car exhaust did decrease between 1968 and 1984, from 698 to 511. Too few data points exist to permit a rigorous statistical analysis, but the graph in Figure 3.3 (for which suicides and accidents have been standardized against a population base for 1968) does, indeed, suggest that the relationship with the "adjusted" measure of cars in operation is closer for accidental deaths than suicides. This provides grounds for believing that some suicides may have circumvented emission controls, with the result that the effect of these controls on the rate of suicide was diminished.

Even if there are grounds for questioning the validity of the "adjusted" measure of cars in operation, there is another possible explanation for the poor fit between this measure and the reduction in car exhaust suicides. This is suggested by the data for Great Britain presented in Figure 3.4, which compares exhaust suicides (standardized against a population base for 1950) with cars in use. There is a close match between the two sets of data until the beginning of the 1970s, when the increase in our exhaust suicides begins to far outstrip the increase in the number of cars.

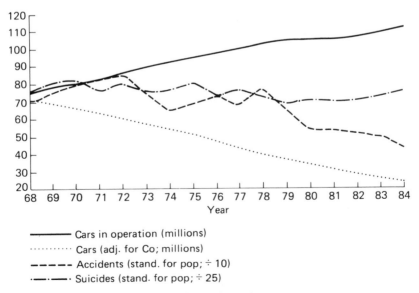

        Cars in operation (millions)
.... Cars (adj. for Co; millions)
– – – –   Accidents (stand. for pop; ÷ 10)
·—·—·   Suicides (stand. for pop; ÷ 25)

Figure 3.3. Car exhaust suicides and accidents, United States, 1968–1984.

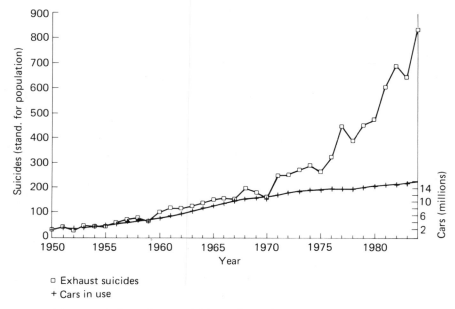

Figure 3.4. Car exhaust suicides and cars in use,
Great Britain, 1950–1984.

Bulusu and Alderson (1984) have suggested that this phenomenon may be
a result of an increase in the number of homes with garages and the increased
popularity of estate and hatchback cars, which require a shorter hose to get
car exhaust into the passenger compartment. Although these kinds of
changes are unlikely to have been sufficient to account for the greatly
increased number of car exhaust suicides, British data to test these ideas are
not readily available.

The more likely explanation, also suggested by Bulusu and Alderson, is
the "snowball" effect of people discovering that this method for suicide is
available. Again, no relevant data are available to test this idea, but it is an
intuitively plausible explanation of the greatly accelerated rate of increase in
the use of this method for suicide. Lester (1987c) has documented the
possibility that publicity of suicides probably increases the rate of suicide
and that there are fashions in the methods chosen for suicide. It is possible,
also, that the snowball effect of increased knowledge might have been given
a "hefty shove" in Britain by the detoxification of domestic gas. Although
little immediate displacement was observed to other methods following
detoxification it is likely that in the longer term populations faced with
reduced opportunities for suicide might gradually seek to expand the
repertoire of alternative methods, especially of those sharing some of the
advantages of those whose availability has been reduced.

A similar phenomenon may have occurred in the United States, namely,
that increased awareness of car exhaust suicides may have led to an increase

in the use of car exhaust at the same time that emission controls were making suicide more difficult with this method. Some support for this idea is provided by Figure 3.5, which shows the rates of car exhaust suicides per million cars in use in Britain and per million "adjusted" cars in the United States.

It can be seen that the two curves are highly correlated (Pearson $r = 0.93$; $p < 0.01$), which suggests that the increases in both countries may have a similar cause. If this is a result of increased knowledge about this method of suicide, the further question arises as to why this occurred at roughly the same time in both countries. An analysis of publicity about suicide during this period in both countries might shed some light on this.

Accepting that emission controls in the United States appear to have reduced the number of car exhaust suicides, the question is how much displacement occurred. Unfortunately, this cannot be answered with any certainty because car exhaust suicides in the United States constituted only a small proportion (about 10 percent) of the total suicides and, between 1960 and 1984, the annual number of suicides increased by 65 percent (from 19,041 to 29,286). This allows ample scope for displacement, but, given the particular advantages of car exhaust poisoning as a method of death (particularly ease and lack of pain), it is unlikely that any such displacement was complete.

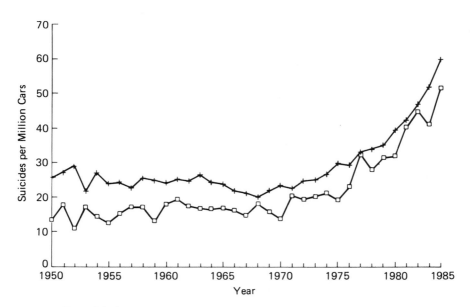

□ Great Britain
+ U.S. (adj. for CO)

Figure 3.5. Car exhaust suicides per million cars, Great Britain and United States, 1950–1984.

A final issue raised by the findings of this study concerns the question of why the ratio of car exhaust suicides to cars in use should, until the advent of emission controls, have been so much greater in the United States than in Britain, even though the overall rates of suicide did not differ much between the two countries (with a rate of 9.8 per 100,000 per year in the United States in 1965 and 9.6 in Britain).

Part of the explanation may lie in differences in such factors as the number of garages or the mean toxicities of car exhausts in the two countries. Perhaps more likely, the difference reflects the disparity in car ownership between the two countries, which, though still considerable (with one car in the United States for every 2.1 people in 1984 compared with one car for every 3.4 people in the Britain), was much greater in 1950 (one car per 4.2 people in the United States compared with one car per 21.8 in the Britain). Any single American citizen therefore had greater access to a car, which may have increased the probability that this method for suicide would be selected. Related to this is the much greater salience of the automobile in the cultural consciousness and way of life, and thus possibly the way of death, of the average American citizen.

In conclusion, the results of this study extend those of the regional study reported earlier and support the idea that emission controls have brought about a decrease in suicide by car exhaust gases in the United States. In Great Britain, where emission controls have yet to be introduced, the rate of suicide by car exhaust has greatly increased in recent years, possibly as a result of increased knowledge about this method for suicide. The British rate, as expressed per million of the population, is now much higher than in the United States, though for many years previously it was much lower.

Conclusions

The studies presented in this chapter support the underlying hypothesis of this volume. The use of car exhaust for suicide is related to the availability of cars (in absolute numbers and per capita) and to their toxicity. The more cars available to people and the more toxic the exhausts, the more likely people are to use car exhaust for suicide.

However, for much of the period studied the use of car exhaust was not a common method for suicide. Therefore, changes in the frequency of use of car exhaust for suicide did not have a detectable effect on the overall suicide rate. The exception to this is in Great Britain in the 1980s, when dramatic increases in car exhaust suicides were associated with the increasing overall suicide rate.

Also equivocal in the results of these car exhaust studies is the question of whether people will switch from one method of suicide to another if the former is made less available. As noted in the previous chapter, suicide by car exhaust is similar in many ways to suicide by domestic gas, which means that switching between these methods might be expected. However, not everyone has equal access to both methods and, at the societal level of analysis, it is very difficult to determine whether the increase in the use of a method for suicide is because the method appeals to a group who would not otherwise have committed suicide or because it encourages suicidal people to switch methods.

Further data on this question of displacement is presented in the next chapter, which deals with the relationship between the availability of firearms and suicide rates.

—— 4 ——

Firearm Availability and Suicide

The role of firearms in violent crime has been a longstanding concern of criminologists International comparisons strongly suggest that the high rates of homicide in the United States are largely attributable to widespread gun ownership (Zimring and Hawkins, 1987). Guns also play a part in much other violent crime. They enable robbers to attack defended targets and are a major cause of robbery killings in the United States.

The role of firearms has also been a concern in accidental death and, of relevance to us, in suicide. For example, Farmer and Rohde (1980) found great variation among nations in the use of firearms for suicide. Setting the standard mortality ratio (SMR) for the suicide rate by firearms at 100 for England and Wales, they found that, although Eire and the Netherlands (both with low ownership of guns) also had low SMRs (0 and 25, respectively), other nations with more freely available guns had much higher ratios; for example, France had an SMR of 836, Australia of 1185, and the United States of 5718.

Farmer and Rohde argued that these results supported the thesis that easy availability and firearms (and other lethal agents) has an important impact on suicide mortality in different nations. Their results certainly lend weight to the suggestion that much of the recent increase in the suicide rate for the United States (from 10.5 per 100,000 per year in 1959 to 12.4 in 1984) is due to an increase in the availability of firearms, at least as measured by firearms manufactured and imported (Boor, 1981; Boyd, 1983). This suggestion is further supported by the fact that the increase in the suicide rate is confined to suicides by firearms. This can be seen from Table 4.1, which shows the changes in the suicide rate by firearms and by all other methods from 1959 to 1984.

It can be seen in the table that the use of firearms has risen steadily since 1959 while the use of other methods for suicide has actually dropped, especially in the 1980s. This is reflected in the changes that have occurred in both the *rates* and the *proportions* of suicides by firearms. The suicide rate by firearms rose from 4.7 in 1959 to 7.2 in 1984, a 53 percent increase. During the same period, the suicide rate by all other methods dropped from 5.8 to

Table 4.1. Gun and nongun suicides in the United States, 1959–1984.

	Suicide rates per 100,00 per year			Percentage of suicides by firearms	
	Total	By gun	Nongun	Males	Females
1959	10.5	4.7	5.8	53.7	24.7
1960	10.5	5.0	5.5	54.2	25.3
1961	10.3	4.7	5.7	54.6	25.2
1962	10.8	5.1	5.7	54.4	25.0
1963	11.0	5.1	5.9	54.0	24.2
1964	10.7	5.1	5.6	55.7	25.4
1965	11.1	5.1	6.0	54.6	23.9
1966	10.8	5.3	5.5	57.0	27.7
1967	10.7	5.3	5.4	57.7	29.1
1968	10.6	5.4	5.2	59.0	30.6
1969	11.0	5.6	5.5	59.2	29.4
1970	11.3	5.7	5.7	58.4	30.2
1971	11.6	5.9	5.7	59.1	32.0
1972	11.9	6.4	5.6	61.1	34.5
1973	11.9	6.3	5.6	61.1	32.2
1974	12.0	6.7	5.3	63.5	35.7
1975	12.5	6.9	5.6	62.1	36.1
1976	12.3	6.8	5.6	62.2	35.5
1977	13.0	7.3	5.7	63.2	36.2
1978	12.3	6.9	5.3	63.6	36.0
1979	12.1	6.9	5.2	63.7	38.0
1980	11.8	6.8	5.0	63.1	38.6
1981	12.0	7.0	5.0	64.3	40.7
1982	12.2	7.1	5.0	64.2	40.7
1983	12.1	7.1	5.0	64.1	40.6
1984	12.4	7.2	5.1	64.0	39.6

5.1, a 12 percent decrease. The percentage of people using firearms for suicide in 1984 rose from 53.7 percent in 1959 to 64.0 percent for men while for women it rose from 24.7 to 39.6 percent. Thus, firearms were clearly used more by both sexes as a method for suicide during this period.

Other research suggests a link between gun availability and suicide; Markush and Bartolucci (1984) compared the suicide rates of the nine major geographic regions of the United States (New England, Middle Atlantic, East North Central, West North Central, South Atlantic, East South Central, West South Central, Mountain, and Pacific). Using survey data from Gallup and the National Opinion Research Center on the extent of gun ownership in each of these regions, they found that gun ownership was associated with the total suicide rate and the firearm suicide rate, but not with the nonfirearm suicide rate. Markush and Bartolucci also found that focusing on the ownership of *handguns* produced a similar but slightly stronger pattern of results. (They did not, however, look at the associations between suicide rates and the ownership of rifles or shotguns.)

The existing research suggests, therefore, that gun ownership may be related to both the firearm suicide rate and the total suicide rate. We have explored these relationships in a number of studies described in this and the next chapter. In the next chapter, we deal with studies of *gun control*, and in this chapter we report on a series of four studies to explore whether differences in the *availability of firearms* are related to the gun suicide rate and possibly to the overall suicide rate.

Studies 6 and 7 examine variations in gun availability and suicide rates among the different states of America. Since no direct measures of the extent of gun ownership for each state exist, availability had to be estimated on the basis of indirect measures. (Incidentally, the U.S. Census Bureau has rejected the suggestion of including questions concerning gun ownership in the 1990 census.) Study 8 examines the relationships between suicide rates and gun ownership for the major regions of the United States and Australia, using household survey measures of ownership. Study 9 also uses household surveys of gun ownership in a time series design to examine the relationship between gun ownership and suicide in the United States between 1959 to 1984.

Suicide and Estimates of Gun Availability in the United States
Study 6

For this comparison of the individual states of America, we decided to follow a suggestion of Linden and Hale (1972) and use the death rate from firearm accidents as an indirect measure of firearm availability. It seemed likely that, in a region where firearm ownership is high, the rate of death from accident with firearms would also be high (McDowall and Loftin, 1985). Although in recent years the accidental death rate from firearms has dropped in America, possibly as a result of changing patterns of ownership of types of firearms or of increased emphasis on adequate training in firearm safety for users, there is no reason to suspect the existence of regional variations in the concern for safety or the establishment of safety training programs for firearm users.[1]

For our second measure, we followed a suggestion by Cook (1982), who in his criminologicl research used the percentage of crimes committed with a gun as a measure of the availability of guns, producing results that make good sense and lend credibility to his measure. The present study therefore used the

---

[1] Research by Lester and Clarke (in preparation) using the data set of Study 9 has shown that the *accidental* death rate from firearms is strongly related to the ownership of *shotguns*.

Table 4.2. Pearson correlation coefficients between measures of gun availability and suicide rates for the states of the United States, 1970.

	Total suicide rate	Suicide rate by guns	Suicide rate by other means
Accidental death rate from guns	0.12	0.54[a]	−0.52[a]
Percentage of homicides by guns	0.05	0.35[a]	−0.38[a]

[a] One-tailed $p < 0.01$.

proportion of homicides in each state committed with a gun as a second indirect measure of firearm availability.

We examined the relationship between these two measures of gun availability and the suicide rates of the 48 continental states for the year 1970. We used the *Vital Statistics of the United States, 1970* to obtain the suicide rates by gun, by all other means and overall for each continental state, the proportion of homicides by guns, and the accidental death rate from guns.

The results can be seen in Table 4.2, where it is clear that both measures of gun availability correlated significantly with the suicide rate by guns. The less available guns were in a state, the lower the suicide rate by guns was. Interestingly, the reduced availability of firearms was related to higher rates of suicide by all other methods. This raises the possibility—discussed at several points later—that there is some switching, or displacement, between methods, depending on availability of guns.

A Further Attempt to Estimate Gun Availability
Study 7

As no direct measures of firearm availability exist for each state, we decided to explore other ways of estimating availability than those used in Study 6. If these alternative measures produced the same results, we could place more confidence in the conclusions.

It seemed possible that the more people who own guns in a state, the higher the per capita subscription to magazines about guns would be. We were not able to locate other research that had used magazine subscriptions as a social indicator, and it is possible, of course, that subscriptions to gun magazines are influenced by factors other than ownership of guns. However, the use of magazine circulations seemed to merit examination. If our predictions were confirmed, the research would support both our thesis and the use of gun magazine subscriptions as a measure of gun ownership.

The Audit Bureau of Circulations provided the circulation of three magazines for firearm owners for 1980: *Shooting Times, Guns & Ammo,* and *American Handgunner.* We obtained rates of suicide and homicide for firearms and other methods from the *Vital Statistics of the United States, 1980.*

Table 4.3 shows the results. States with higher per capita circulations of the three gun magazines had higher suicide rates by firearm but not different suicide rates by all other methods. However, the overall suicide rate was higher in those states with the higher firearm magazine circulations. Thus, the selective associations in these results suggest that the per capita circulation of firearm magazines is specifically related to suicides by firearms. It does appear that, if the circulation of firearm magazines is a valid index of gun ownership, the availability of guns may by related to their increased use for suicide and to a higher overall suicide rate.

Some of the results of this study are consistent with those from the previous study using other indirect measures of firearm availability. In both studies, the measures of gun availability were associated with the *firearm suicide rate.* However, although the accidental death rate from firearms and the percentage of homicides by guns (Study 6) correlated negatively with the *suicide rate by other means,* the per capita circulations of gun magazines did not.

Reasons for these discrepancies are not easy to discover. Interpretation of the studies is complicated by the fact that, because they were undertaken separately they used suicide data for different time periods. Moreover, the lack of state-level measures of actual gun ownership, which forced us to use indirect measures of availability, means that no good criteria exist against which to validate our measures. However, we can begin to place some confidence in a result that is repeated, whatever the measure of gun availability: firearm availability does indeed appear to be associated with the suicide rate by firearms.

Table 4.3. Correlations between firearm magazine subscriptions and suicide rates for the states of the United States, 1980.

Suicide rate	Shooting Times	Guns and Ammo	American Handgunner
Overall	0.56^a	0.47^a	0.40^b
By firearm	0.58^a	0.55^a	0.38^b
By other means	0.10	−0.01	0.13

[a] One-tailed $p < 0.001$
[b] One-tailed $p < 0.01$.

A Comparison of the United States and Australia
Study 8

The two previous studies examined the relationship between estimates of gun availability in the individual states of the United States and the use of guns for suicide. Recent household surveys in Australia have produced figures for the extent of gun ownership in the different states there. The present study explores whether gun ownership is related to the suicide rate in those states and compares the results with those found for the major regions of the United States. Household survey data about gun ownership similar to that for Australia does exist for America, though only at the regional and not the state level.

We obtained data for the percentage of households with guns, the overall suicide rates, and the percentage of suicides by gun for six of the seven Australian states from Harding (1981). Data from the seventh, Northern Territories, were incomplete and could not be used. We obtained death rates for the regions of the United States from the *Vital Statistics of the United States, 1970* and regional data on gun ownership from Wright et al. (1983).

Table 4.4 presents the associations and compares the results from Australia with those from the United States.

The percentage of households in which guns are owned in the Australian states was strongly related to the percentage of suicides by guns (Pearson $r = 0.87$ for males, $p < 0.05$). The percentage of households with guns was related positively to the suicide rate by guns ($r = 0.68$), negatively to the suicide rate by other means ($r = -0.79$, $p < 0.05$), but only weakly to the overall suicide rate ($r = 0.29$).[2]

Despite the difference between the two countries in the use of guns for suicide (35 percent of suicides in Australia in 1975–1977 versus 55 percent for the United States in the same period), a similar pattern of results was found for the nine major regions of the United States; that is, areas with higher rates of gun ownership had higher suicide rates by gun and slightly lower suicide rates by all other means.

Even if their import is lessened by the small number of states covered in the Australian data and regions covered in the American data, these results are important because we used actual measures of gun ownership. They support the results of Study 6, which used gun homicides and gun accidents as indirect measures of gun availability in the states. Also, like those of Study 6 (but not of Study 7), these results imply displacement in that higher levels of gun ownership are not associated with higher total suicide rates;

---

[2] The correlations using the number of guns per capita were not as strong as those using the percentage of households possessing a gun, but they gave a similar pattern of results.

Table 4.4. Correlations between gun ownership and suicide rates in Australia and the United States.

	Australia, 1975 (6 states)		United States, 1970 (9 regions)
	Guns/capita	Percentage of households with guns	Guns/capita
Suicide rate	0.31	0.29	0.22
Suicide rate by firearm	0.47[a]	0.68[a]	0.83[c]
Suicide rate by other means	− 0.42[a]	− 0.79[a,b]	− 0.52
Percentage suicides by firearms	0.56[a]	0.87[a]	0.93[c]

[a] Data were available for males only for these correlations.
[b] One-tailed $p < 0.05$.
[c] One-tailed $p < 0.01$.

rather, they are associated with a higher firearm suicide rate and a lower suicide rate by all other methods.

We will discuss this issue of displacement in more detail in Chapter 6. For now, we should note that strong evidence has been provided that the geographic variation in availability of firearms is related to their use for suicide. This has been done for the states of America using various indices of firearm ownership, and it has been confirmed for the large regions of the United States and the states of Australia by more direct measures of firearm ownership.

The complementary question we have to answer is whether variations in firearm ownership *over time* are also related to their use for suicide. This question is addressed by the next study in our series.

Gun Ownership in the United States and Suicide Rates from 1959 to 1984
Study 9

As mentioned previously, a number of commentators have suggested that the increase in suicide in the United States over the past 25 years could be a result of the increased availability of guns, at least as measured by the number of guns manufactured domestically and imported. However, this increase in the *number* of guns has not resulted in the wider *ownership* of firearms: surveys undertaken in the 1980s show that about 45 percent of all households owned a gun, which if anything, is a somewhat lower percentage than that of 25 years earlier (Wright et al., 1983). The lack of increase in household ownership is explained by the fact that the growing number of guns has been accompanied by an increased number of households and also, apparently, by greater number of guns per gun-owning households (Wright et al., 1983).

This lack of increase in household ownership of guns would create substantial difficulties for the gun availability hypothesis were it not for changes in patterns of ownership. As will be seen later, the surveys indicate that, although household ownership of rifles has not altered and ownership of shotguns has declined (possibly because a greater proportion of new households are female-headed and are in urban and metropolitan areas), handgun ownership has increased substantially, possibly because of increased fear of crime and the perceived need for self-protection (Wright et al., 1983). The increase in the U.S. suicide rate might therefore be due, not to an increase of guns in general but to an increase only in the availability of *handguns*.

In support of this narrower hypothesis, it should be noted that the ecological fit between the distribution of gun ownership and suicide in the nine major regions of the United States is closer when ownership only of handguns is considered (Markush and Bartolucci, 1984). Three studies (Danto, 1972; Browning, 1974a; Wintemute et al., 1988) have also shown that, relative to their numbers, handguns are more likely to be used for suicide than rifles or shotguns, though in each case samples were taken only from local areas and, except in the most recent study, were also small.[3]

Aside from the statistical data, there are a number of a priori reasons for expecting handguns to be more implicated in suicide:

---

[3] More comprehensive but still inadequate data from the U.S. *Vital Statistics* (which in 1979 began to publish figures for the guns used in suicide) suggest handguns play a lesser but important part. In 1984, for example, almost as many cases of suicide with handguns were recorded as with other guns even though more households had rifles and shotguns. However, in only 37 percent of gun suicides was the type of gun specified; had records been more complete, the disproportionate representation of handguns might have proved much greater. This is suggested by a comparison of homicide data for 1984 in the *Vital Statistics* and the FBI *Crime Reports*. In the former, only 8 percent gun homicides are shown as having been committed with a handgun, whereas about 12 percent involved shooting with a rifle or shotgun. (In the remaining 80 percent the gun was not specified.) In the FBI reports (which failed to specify gun type in only 6 percent of cases) 74 percent of gun homicides are recorded as having been committed with a handgun and 20 percent with some other gun. This comparison between the two data sources shows substantially more underrecording in the *Vital Statistics* of the use of handguns in homicide than of the use of other guns. The same may be true of suicides, and possibly for similar reasons: suicides and homicides, when commited with a shotgun or rifle, not only may be more unusual but may result in more damage to the body. The medical examiner may therefore be more likely in these cases to record the type of gun used. (It appears, however, that *Vital Statistics* is classifying an increasing number of gun suicides each year by gun type.)

1. they are easier to use for this purpose (Hirsh, 1960),
2. they are less likely to disfigure (which may be especially important for women),
3. they are more likely to be kept loaded and at hand for self-protection, and
4. they have a stronger cultural association as personal rather than hunting or sporting weapons (Tonso, 1982), and hence may be more readily turned against oneself.

The present study therefore investigates the following hypothesis: that the increase in the rate of both gun suicides and all suicides between 1959 and 1984 is closely related to the increase in household ownership of handguns.

Data Sources and Method

We obtained data concerning suicide for 1959–1984 from the annual volumes of the *Vital Statistics of the United States*. This source provided annual counts of both suicide in general and suicides by firearms and explosives. About 98 percent of the latter category are gun suicides (Newton and Zimring, 1969). We obtained numbers of households and mean household size for 1959–1984 from the annual editions of the *Statistical Abstract of the United States* for generating annual estimates of the population used in calculating suicide rates.

We obtained data on the proportion of households with guns from opinion polls conducted by Gallup in 1959, 1965, 1968, 1972, 1975, and 1983 and by the National Opinion Research Center in 1973, 1974, 1976, 1977, 1980, 1982, and 1984. In all cases, the samples consisted of about 1500 respondents selected to be representative of the total adult population of the continental United States who are noninstitutionalized and English-speaking. One person in each household was interviewed.

To deal with the problem of missing data on gun ownership for 13 of the 26 years in the period studied, four techniques were used: the years with missing data were ignored; a missing year was allowed to take the value of the previous year with data; a missing year was allowed to take the value of the next year with data; and missing years were allowed to take a value consistent with a smooth trend between adjacent years with data. Results from all four techniques gave similar results, and only results from the last method are reported here.

Results

It can be seen from Table 4.1 (presented earlier) that the rate of gun suicides per 100,000 has increased by more than 50 percent (from 4.7 in 1959 to 7.2 in 1984), while a small decline in the rate of nongun suicides has occurred. Indeed, the increase in the overall suicide rate is accounted for entirely by the increase in gun suicides.

As for trends in firearm ownership, it is evident from Table 4.5 that, although little change occurred overall in the proportion of households with a gun during the period, there were important changes in the kinds of gun owned. The proportion of households with long guns declined, which was offset by a considerable rise in the proportion of households with handguns (from 16 percent in 1959 to 21 percent in 1984). Together with a marked increase in the number of households, this resulted in almost a doubling of the number of households with handguns during the period, from an estimated 8.2 million in 1959 (that is, 16 percent of 51,302,000) to 17.9 million in 1984 (21 percent of 85,407,000).

The close relationship between the increases in the number of gun suicides and the number of handgun households is suggested by the graph in Figure 4.1.

For the regression analysis, the dependent variable was the incidence of suicide calculated as the number of suicides per 100,000 households. The independent variable was the percentage of households with access to a gun.

Regressing the total suicide rates for the United States on each of the four measures of gun ownership (Table 4.6) produced no significant coefficients (P was set at .001 because of the small number of cases and the need to difference data because of autocorrelation), and separate analyses for the suicide rates of males and females produced similar results.

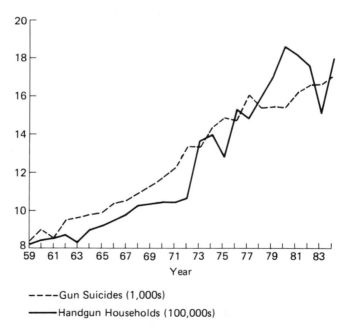

Figure 4.1. Gun suicides and handgun households, United States, 1959–1984.

Table 4.5. U.S. households with guns, 1959–1984.

Year	Households (1000's)	Percentage of households owning			
		Guns	Handguns	Rifles	Shotguns
1959	51,302	49	16	27	32
1960[a]	52,799	49.83	16	26.5	32.17
1961[a]	53,464	48.66	16	26	32.34
1962[a]	54,652	48.49	16	25.5	32.51
1963[a]	55,189	48.32	16	25	32.68
1964[a]	55,996	48.15	16	24.5	32.85
1965	57,436	48	16	24	33
1966[a]	58,092	48.67	16.33	27.33	33
1967[a]	58,845	49.33	16.67	30.67	33
1968	60,444	50	17	34	33
1969[a]	61,805	48.25	16.75	32	31.5
1970[a]	63,401	46.50	16.5	30	30
1971[a]	64,374	44.75	16.25	28.5	28.5
1972	66,676	43	16	26	27
1973	68,251	47	20	29	27
1974	69,859	46	20	27	28
1975	71,120	44	18	26	26
1976	72,867	46	21	28	28
1977	74,142	50	20	30	31
1978[a]	76,030	49	21	29.67	30.33
1979[a]	77,330	48	22	29.33	29.67
1980	80,776	47	23	29	29
1981[a]	82,368	46	22	28.5	28.5
1982	83,527	45	21	28	28
1983	83,918	40	18	25	24
1984	85,407	45	21	27	28

[a] Figures are interpolated for gun ownership.

Table 4.6. Regression analyses of all suicides and gun suicides[a] for the data in tables 4.1 and 4.5 (for the United States, 1959–1984).

	Unstandardized b	SE	Beta	P
All suicides				
Handgun	− .003	.001	− 0.417	0.038
Rifle	− .001	.001	− 0.225	0.278
Shotgun	.001	.001	0.078	0.709
All guns	.000	.001	0.041	0.846
Gun suicides				
Handgun	.004	.001	0.684	0.001
Rifle	− .000	.001	− 0.089	0.672
Shotgun	.001	.001	0.136	0.834
All guns	.000	.001	0.044	0.518

[a] With the exception of gun suicides regressed on handgun availability, each of the time series had significant serial correlation (identified by the Durbin–Watson statistic). Each of the serially correlated series was differenced and reanalyzed, and in each case first-order differencing removed the serial correlation. In addition, plots of expected values and residuals were examined for possible heteroscedasticity. No such problems were evident.

Regressing the gun suicide rate for the United States produced one significant positive coefficient, namely, with handgun availability (see Table 4.6). This relationship appeared to be a little stronger for male gun suicide rates than for female gun suicide rates.

Discussion

As expected the regression analysis demonstrated a strong correlation between increases in handgun ownership and the rate of gun suicides, and thus provides further reason to think that the relationship may be causal. The fact that no significant correlation was found between the increased availability of handguns and the rise in the overall rate of suicide, however, leaves the important question of displacement unresolved. Increased handgun availability may lead, not to an increase in suicide, but merely to the increased use of guns by people who would otherwise have used some other method. According to this interpretation, the overall increase in suicide is the result of a general rise in suicidal motivation, in which case reducing the availability of handguns would result not in a reduction of suicide, but only a return to other methods.

However, there is no independent evidence of an increase in suicidal motivation, which could just as easily have remained stable or fallen. In either of these latter cases the failure of the regression analysis to demonstrate a relationship between handgun availability and the overall rate of suicide could be attributed to the fact that nongun suicides had not only declined by the end of the period but had fluctuated throughout. Their inclusion in the overall rate of suicide thus dilutes the correlation with increased availability of handguns.

Conclusions

This chapter has reported research showing higher rates of suicide by firearms in those parts of the United States and Australia where guns are more widely available. In addition, a time-series study showed that the increased availability of *handguns* was strongly associated with the increase in *gun* suicides in the United States.

Given the orientation of this volume, these results were largely expected, and they support the general thesis that suicide might be prevented by restricting the availability of lethal agents. However, it was not clear from the studies reported whether the increased availability of guns serves to raise the overall rate of suicide or merely to displace the choice of method so that people already intent on suicide would be more likely to use a gun. The results of the time-series analysis reported in Study 9 were equivocal on this matter, as were those of the regional analyses reported in Studies 6 through 8. In Study 6, states with more guns (as measured by gun accident deaths and the percentage of homicides with guns) and more gun suicides were found to have lower rates of suicide by all other methods and no higher overall levels of suicide. Similar results supporting displacement were found in Study 8, which examined actual gun ownership in the Australian states and the nine major regions of the United States. However, the state-level data for firearm magazine subscriptions in the United States (Study 7) did not support displacement; higher subscription rates to firearm magazines were related to both higher rates of gun suicide and higher overall rates of suicide.

Whether increased availability of guns results in either higher rates of suicide or displacement is crucial to the debate about prevention. The question can be answered only through the collection of better data, and it is important that the *Vital Statistics* improves its records of the kind of guns used in suicide. Much more accurate data are also needed concerning gun ownership. At present, this is only crudely measured on a regional basis, it can only be estimated at the state level, and no data at all exist at the individual level. It is to be hoped that the Census Bureau can be persuaded to include questions on gun ownership in the 2000 census even if they have rejected this for 1990.

In the meantime, sample surveys would help to fill the gap. Not only might these provide more reliable measurement at the state level, but they might also provide much useful information on usage and attitudes. They might enquire how and why guns are obtained, whether legally, where they are kept, and which members of the household have use of them or access to them. Such questions should be supplemented by deeper probing of attitudes (of both men and women and for different age groups) toward the use of guns for suicide and the alternatives that might be considered were guns less readily available (see Chapters 6 and 7). Only when information of this kind is available will it be possible to predict with any confidence the consequences of increasing or decreasing levels of gun ownership.

——5——

Handgun Control Statutes

Chapter 4 provided good evidence that the availability of firearms. especially handguns, has an impact on the suicide rate by firearms, and possibly on the overall suicide rate. It seems possible, therefore, that *restricting* the availability of handguns through limitations on purchasing and ownership might also reduce the suicide rate by guns (see Danto, 1979; Sim, 1979). If no more than a few of those who would have used guns for suicide switch to other methods, then states with the strictest gun control laws may have lower overall rates of suicide.

Rules governing the selling, purchasing, and carrying of guns in the United States vary from state to state. This "within-nation" variation permits an analysis of the relationship between the strictness of gun control laws and the rates of suicide. Do states with the strictest gun control laws have the lowest suicide rates?

In this chapter we report a series of studies on the relationship between handgun control laws and suicide rates that supports this conclusion.

Earlier Research on Gun Control Laws

The early research on the impact of strict gun control laws was conducted primarily to explore whether strict gun control laws had any impact on violent crime, especially murder (for example, Seitz, 1972; Murray, 1975). Only an occasional study included suicide as a dependent variable.

The first such study was conducted by Geisel et al. (1969), who quantified the strictness of state handgun control laws by weighting the various characteristics of the laws to achieve the strongest association with violent crime rates—a questionable procedure since it biases the study in favor of the authors' hypothesis. They calculated correlations for both states and cities (in 1960 and 1965); finding a negative association, they concluded that strict handgun control laws did reduce the homicide rates, the suicide rates, and the rates of accidental deaths by firearms. Strict handgun control laws had no impact on robberies or aggravated assaults.

Medoff and Magaddino (1983) explored correlates of the white male suicide rate over the American states in 1970. In a multiple regression analysis, they found that the requirement of a license to purchase a gun and a required waiting period between purchase and delivery was negatively associated with the suicide rate and helped explain the variability of the suicide rate. Suicide rates for white males were also lower in the six states with the strictest gun control laws (Hawaii, Michigan, Missouri, New Jersey, New York, and North Carolina).[1]

Coding and Scaling the Gun Laws

In this chapter, we present a series of studies analyzing the relationship between handgun control laws in the continental United States and both firearm suicide rates and the overall suicide rate. In most of these studies we used data from Bakal (1968), who coded the handgun control laws in each state for eight characteristics:

1. Is a license or permit required to purchase a handgun?
2. Is a waiting period required between the purchase and the delivery of the handgun?
3. Are handgun sales reported to the police?
4. Is a license required to sell handguns at retail?
5. Is there a minimum age requirement for buying or receiving a handgun?
6. Is a permit or license required to own a handgun (to keep at home or at a place of business)?
7. Is a permit or license required to carry a handgun openly on one's person.
8. Is a permit or license required to carry a handgun concealed on one's person.

A visual inspection of the codes indicated that a Guttman scale for measuring strictness could be constructed using seven of the eight characteristics. A Guttman scale is one in which the characteristics can be ordered in such a way that if a state has characteristic $(n + 1)$, it will also have characteristic n (but not necessarily vice versa). The Guttman scale is shown in Table 5.1. Setting the "some" ratings as "yes" ratings produced a Guttman scale with a coefficient of reproducibility of 0.95 and a coefficient of scalability of 0.79.

---

[1] The study by Medoff and Magaddino appeared in print after the publication of some of the earlier accounts of the research reported in this chapter by the present authors. Our studies have not been presented in this book in the order in which they were carried out and published, but rather in an order that provides a coherent organization for the book.

Table 5.1. Guttman scale for measuring the strictness of gun control laws.

State	Minimum age >18	License to carry a concealed gun prohibited	License to sell a gun	Sales reported to police	Waiting period to collect	License to buy a gun	License to own a gun
7 IL	Y	Y	Y	Y	Y	Y	Y
NY	Y	Y	Y	Y	Y	Y	Y
6 MA	Y	Y	Y	Y	Y	Y	N
MI	Y	Y	Y	Y	Y	Y	N
NJ	Y	Y	Y	Y	Y	Y	N
NC	Y	Y	Y	N	Y	Y	N
MO	Y	Y	N	Y	Y	Y	N
5 AL	Y	Y	Y	Y	Y	N	N
CA	Y	Y	Y	Y	Y	N	N
CT	Y	Y	Y	Y	Y	N	N
MD	Y	Y	Y	Y	Y	N	N
PA	Y	Y	Y	Y	Y	N	N
RI	Y	Y	Y	Y	Y	N	N
WA	Y	Y	Y	Y	Y	N	N
TN	Y	N	Y	Y	Y	N	N
IN	Y	Y	Y	N	Y	N	N
SD	Y	Y	Y	N	Y	N	N
4 DE	Y	Y	Y	Y	N	N	N
IA	Y	Y	Y	Y	N	N	N
WV	Y	Y	Y	Y	N	N	N
GA	Y	Y	Y	S	N	N	N
ND	Y	Y	S	Y	N	N	N
OR	Y	Y	S	Y	N	N	N
VA	Y	Y	S	S	N	N	N
KY	Y	Y	N	S	N	N	N
3 LA	Y	Y	Y	N	N	N	N
SC	Y	Y	Y	N	N	N	N
TX	Y	Y	Y	N	N	N	N
NH	Y	N	Y	N	N	N	N
2 AZ	Y	Y	N	N	N	N	N
FL	Y	Y	N	N	N	N	N
ID	Y	Y	N	N	N	N	N
KS	Y	Y	N	N	N	N	N
NE	Y	Y	N	N	N	N	N
MS	Y	Y	N	N	N	N	N
MT	Y	Y	N	N	N	N	N
ME	Y	Y	N	N	N	N	N
NV	Y	Y	N	N	N	N	N
OH	Y	Y	N	N	N	N	N
OK	Y	Y	N	N	N	N	N
UT	Y	Y	N	N	N	N	N
WI	Y	Y	N	N	N	N	N

Table 5.1. (Continued)

State	Minimum age >18	License to carry a concealed gun prohibited a	License to sell a gun	Sales reported to police	Waiting period to collect	License to buy a gun	License to own a gun
WY	Y	Y	N	N	N	N	N
CO	N	Y	N	N	N	N	N
1 MN	Y	N	N	N	N	N	N
VT	Y	N	N	N	N	N	N
0 AR	N	N	N	N	N	N	N
NM	N	N	N	N	N	N	N

^{a} Abbreviations:
  Y = yes
  N = no
  S = some municipalities

Handgun Control and Deaths from Suicide
Study 10

In this study, we explored the relationship between the measure of the strictness of state handgun control laws in 1968 and death rates from suicide in 1960 and 1970 based on data obtained from the *Vital Statistics of the United States* for 1960 and 1970. We examined the relationship between the strictness of state handgun control laws and the *absolute* death rates in 1960 and 1970. We also looked at the *changes* in these rates during this decade to see if strict handgun control laws had a continuing and cumulative impact on the suicide rates. We looked at the total suicide rate and also at the rates for each method of suicide.

Table 5.2 shows correlations between the strictness of the handgun control laws and suicide rates. It can be seen that states with the stricter handgun control laws had lower rates of suicide by firearms, in both 1960 (Pearson $r = -0.46$) and 1970 ($r = -0.52$). The strictness of the state handgun control laws was not related to the rates of suicides by poisons or by hanging/strangulation. States with stricter handgun control laws had higher rates of suicide by "other" means, which once again suggests that, to some extent, a reduced availability of one method for suicide may induce some people to switch to other methods. However, the finding that the total suicide rate was lower in the states with the stricter handgun control laws indicates that only a few suicidal people may switch to an alternative method.

We checked these results for the preventive effects of strict handgun control laws on suicide rates for each age group in the United States. For

Table 5.2. Correlations between the strictness of the handgun control laws and suicide rates.

	1960	1970	Change from 1960 to 1970
Total suicide rate	-0.24^a	-0.41^b	-0.35^b
Male suicide rate	-0.29^a	-0.49^b	-0.23^a
Female suicide rate	0.01	-0.15	-0.32^a
Suicide due to			
poisons	-0.01	-0.07	-0.10
hanging/strangulation	0.23	0.15	-0.20
firearms	-0.46^b	-0.52^b	-0.23
other means	0.34^b	0.43^b	-0.11
Proportion of suicides by firearms	-0.45^b	-0.44^b	0.02

[a] One-tailed $p<0.05$.
[b] One-tailed $p<0.01$.

1970, the negative correlation between strict handgun control laws and a lower overall suicide rate was found for the suicide rate of each age group of the population: $r = -0.35$ for those aged 15 to 24, -0.33 for those aged 25 to 34, -0.29 for those aged 35 to 44, -0.47 for those aged 45 to 54, -0.40 for those aged 55 to 64, and -0.27 for those 65 years of age and older. The consistency of these results shows that age is not a confounding variable in the association between strict gun control laws and lower suicide rates.

This initial study, therefore, supported the association between the strictness of handgun control laws in a state and both a higher suicide rate by firearms and a higher overall suicide rate. There was evidence for a small amount of switching to the residual methods of suicide in states where handgun control laws were stricter but no evidence of switching to suicide by poisons or by hanging. Thus, the overall rate of suicide was lower in states with the stricter handgun control laws.

Characteristics of the Handgun Laws
Study 11

It may be that the different features of the handgun control statutes are not all associated strongly with the lower suicide rates. Some may be more pertinent than others. To provide a more detailed analysis of the effect of the 1986 handgun control laws on suicide, we coded the handgun control laws for each characteristic provided by Bakal (1968).

It appeared reasonable to assume that statute characteristics could be indicative of several dimensions of restrictiveness. Preliminary analysis of the characteristics lent support to the belief that more than one dimension was present. For example, as we will see later, state legal restrictions on handgun sellers are not always accompanied by restrictions on the purchaser of handguns.

After the statutes for the states were coded, a principal component analysis was used to determine the structure of the statute characteristics.[2]

Table 5.3 presents the rotated factors obtained from the analysis. The three factors derived indicate three distinct dimensions of statute characteristics. An examination of factor I shows high loadings for statute characteristics pertaining to handgun *sales*. Factor II shows high loading for restrictions on *purchases and ownership*. Permits to *carry* a weapon, either openly or concealed, are highly loaded on factor III.

We then examined the relationship between the principal components of handgun control laws (using the factor scores produced by the computer program) and rates of firearm suicide. Table 5.4 presents the zero-order correlations between the components of the handgun control laws and the firearm suicide rates. It is clear that factors I (sales) and II (purchase and ownership) are related to the firearm suicide rate, but the correlation between factor III (carrying weapons) and the firearm suicide rate is very low and not statistically significant. Thus, restrictions on selling and buying handguns appear to be the most important dimensions of the statutes. The negative correlations between factors I and II and suicide rates involving guns are similar for 1960 and 1970.

Table 5.3. A principal component analysis of 1968 state gun control statute characteristics (varimax rotation).

	Factors		
	I	II	III
1. License or permit required to purchase handguns	0.43	0.67[a]	−0.02
2. Waiting period required between purchase and delivery	0.84[a]	0.34	−0.03
3. Handgun sales reported to police	0.70[a]	0.35	0.02
4. License required to sell handguns at retail	0.80[a]	0.14	0.20
5. Minimum age requirement for purchasing (>18 years)	0.71[a]	−0.31	0.27
6. Permit or license required to own handgun	0.07	0.84[a]	0.17
7. Permit or license required to carry handgun openly	0.01	0.41	0.71[a]
8. Permit or license required to carry handgun concealed	0.18	−0.07	0.78
Cumulative percentage of variance (%)	39.5	55.3	68.9

[a] High loading.

---

[2] We used the SPSS FACTOR program with a varimax rotation (Kim, 1975).

Table 5.4. Relation between factor scores and suicide rates.

	Factors		
	I Restrictions on seller	II Restrictions on buyer	III Restrictions on carrier
Percentage of suicides			
Using guns, 1960	-0.39^a	-0.39^a	-0.01
Using guns, 1970	-0.40^a	-0.35^a	-0.03
Using guns, change	-0.03	0.07	-0.04
Rates of suicide			
Poison, 1960	0.09	-0.09	-0.04
Poison, 1970	0.04	-0.10	-0.06
Poison, change	-0.06	-0.05	-0.04
Hanging, 1960	0.19	0.16	-0.08
Hanging, 1970	0.20	0.09	-0.04
Hanging, change	-0.09	-0.14	0.07
Guns, 1960	-0.37^a	-0.40^a	-0.02
Guns, 1970	-0.42^a	-0.40^a	-0.07
Guns, change	-0.19	-0.10	-0.09
Other means, 1960	0.22	0.40^a	-0.01
Other means, 1970	0.34^a	0.23	0.06
Other means, change	-0.05	-0.29^b	0.05

[a] One-tailed $p < 0.01$.
[b] One-tailed $p < 0.05$.

We also examined the relationship between handgun control factor scores and suicides involving guns while controlling for other demographic variables. We obtained data on the percentage of nonwhites, of males, and of young people, and the population density of the states from the *Statistical Abstract of the United States.* Table 5.5 presents the first- through fourth-order partial correlation coefficients with the percentage of suicides involving guns for 1970 as the dependent variable. Although the zero-order correlations are reduced by some of the partial correlations, the relationship between factor I (restrictions on the seller) and suicides involving guns remained negative and significant.

Before any conclusions are drawn from the studies presented so far in this chapter, some caveats are necessary since these findings have limitations.

First, the codings of the state handgun control statutes for each year from 1960 to 1970 (rather than for 1968 alone, as in the present set of studies) would permit an examination of changes in the laws as well as changes in the patterns of personal violence. Second, there is a need to control for additional variables such as region of the United States. Third, there were no measures of the enforcement of the handgun laws or the actual ownership of handguns available for use.

Nevertheless, the research identified some interesting relationships that

Table 5.5. Relationship between gun control law factors and percentage of suicides by guns in 1970, controlling for demographic variables by means of partial correlation coefficients.

	Factors		
	I Restrictions on seller	II Restrictions on buyer	III Restrictions on carrier
Zero order	−0.41[a]	−0.35[b]	−0.05
Controlling for			
percent of black population	−0.53[a]	−0.40[a]	−0.11
percent of male population	−0.37[b]	−0.29	−0.05
population density	−0.13	−0.22	0.05
percent of aged 14–24	−0.37[b]	−0.24	−0.09
percent of blacks and of males	−0.50[a]	−0.25	−0.16
percent of blacks and population density	−0.30[b]	−0.29	−0.03
percent of blacks and of aged 14–24	−0.49[a]	−0.30[b]	−0.14
percent of males and population density	−0.14	−0.24	0.05
percent of males and of aged 14–24	−0.36[b]	−0.23	−0.09
population density and percent of aged 14–24	−0.14	−0.16	0.01
percent of blacks, percent of males, and population density	−0.30[b]	−0.21	−0.06
percent of blacks, of males, and of aged 14–24	−0.48[a]	−0.22	−0.16
percent of blacks, population density, and percent of aged 14–24	−0.29	−0.25	−0.25
percent of males, population density, and percent of aged 14–24	−0.15	−0.20	0.02
percent of blacks, percent of males, population density, and percent of aged 14–24	−0.30[b]	−0.20	−0.07

[a] One-tailed $p < 0.01$.
[b] One-tailed $p < 0.05$.

may provide direction for future studies. The importance of restrictions on retail firearm sales for controlling violent crimes such as homicide and armed robbery has been discussed by Zimring (1975). The present findings suggest that restrictions placed on buyers may also reduce suicides involving guns. Restrictions on *carrying* handguns appeared to be unimportant.

The consistent relationship between suicide rates by guns and handgun control statutes, together with the evidence from other studies that strict handgun control laws have little impact on violent crime rates, may indicate that limiting access to guns is effective for violent acts that result from transient *crisis* situations. For a potential suicide victim, a waiting period for the purchase of a gun may deter the act until the crisis has passed.

It should be noted that the gun control statutes scaled for strictness in these studies were those pertaining to handguns. Future research could investigate the statutes involving other types of guns.

Availability of Guns and Moral Opposition to Suicide
Study 12

We have seen that the availability of guns appears to be related to the suicide rates of the states of the United States. Several investigators have focused on the acceptability of suicide as a solution to problems. Farber (1968) and Jacobs (1982), for example, both argue that suicide is much more likely to be committed by people who find it morally acceptable, as have Dublin and Bunzel (1933) and Henderson and Williams (1974). Most major religions disapprove of suicide and even consider it a major sin. Individual personal philosophies may also see suicide as an unacceptable act. Jacobs (1967) has documented from their suicide notes how suicides try to justify their actions and absolve themselves of blame when they are about to kill themselves. To some extent this variable becomes part of a cycle. If society has a tolerant attitude toward suicide, suicide may well become more common. But then, as suicide becomes more common, the society may become more used to, familiar with, and accepting of suicide.

The present study was designed to test the power of these two variables in predicting regional suicide rates—the availability of a popular method for suicide and the acceptance of suicide as a solution for life's problems.[3]

For the present study, we used the state handgun control laws for the year 1980 with codings of the laws provided by Jones and Ray (1980). Only five characteristics used in the previously discussed research were available from the Jones and Ray Codings: (1) Is a license or permit required to purchase a handgun? (2) Are handgun sales reported to the police? (3) Is a license required to sell handguns at retail? (4) Is a permit or license required to own a handgun (to keep at home or at a place of business)? (5) Is a permit or license required to carry a handgun concealed on one's person? The Pearson correlation between the strictness of the handgun control laws in 1968 from Study 10 and the present codings for 1980 was 0.77.

Since most of the major religions see suicide as an unacceptable act, religiosity was used as a measure of the societal acceptance of suicide. Previous research on religiosity has used poor measures, such as the percentage of Roman Catholics in the society or the percentage of books published that are religious (Stack, 1980). The present study used church

---

[3] We make a distinction here between the acceptability of suicide as a solution to life's problems in general and the acceptability of a particular method for suicide once a person has decided to commit suicide. We return to this latter issue in subsequent chapters.

attendance in each state from a recently published survey of the United States (Quinn et al., 1982). It was felt that church attendance in each state would be a reasonably good measure of the strength of religious views in the states.

We obtained suicide rates for the 48 continental states for 1980 from the *Vital Statistics of the United States, 1980.*

The results are shown in Table 5.6, where it can be seen that suicide rates were lower in states with the stricter handgun control laws and lower in states where church attendance was higher. The correlations between suicide rates and each of the variables remained statistically significant even when the other variable was controlled through the use of partial correlation coefficients. Finally, a multiple correlation between suicide rates and both variables—handgun laws and church attendance—was calculated. This was found to be 0.68, indicating that the two variables together explained 46 percent of the variation in the suicide rates of the states.

Conclusions

The research in the present chapter has shown that firearm availability, as measured by the strictness of state handgun control laws, is strongly related to the suicide rate by firearms and to the overall suicide rate. This one variable, together with church attendance, accounts for 46 percent of the variation in the suicide rates of the states.

These findings are congruent with those in the previous chapter, in which we found that ownership of guns, particularly handguns, was strongly related to their use in suicide. As far as displacement is concerned (the

Table 5.6. Correlations between suicide rates and the strictness of handgun control laws and church attendance in the United States, 1980.

	Suicide rate
Handgun law strictness	-0.57^a
Church attendance	-0.49^a
Partial correlations	
handgun law strictness controlling	
for church attendance	-0.54^a
church attendance controlling	
for handgun laws	-0.45^a
Multiple correlations	
handgun law strictness &	
church attendance	0.68

[a] One-tailed $p < 0.01$.

subject of the next chapter), only the results from Study 10 are relevant. Congruent with Study 7 in the previous chapter, which used the circulation of gun magazines as an index of gun ownership, this showed that the more available guns are, the higher the *total* suicide rate is. Hence, there was no evidence of displacement.

The research reviewed in this chapter raises many issues worthy of further study. The present set of studies focused primarily on handgun statutes in 1968, and it would be useful to replicate these findings for other years. It would be interesting to explore whether *changes* in the handgun control laws was accompanied by changes in the use of firearms for suicide. In particular, weakening of the handgun laws (as in Florida in 1987) might have a powerful impact on suicide rates by increasing the number of handguns owned by citizens. (Strengthening handgun control laws might have a lesser impact because many people might already have bought handguns).

We have mentioned that the existence of handgun control laws does not necessarily imply strict enforcement of the laws. Thus, future research should endeavor to measure and take into account enforcement of the laws (perhaps by counting prosecutions and convictions under the handgun control statutes).

We conclude by noting that many of our studies are correlational and thus, strictly speaking, do not permit causal inferences. To take the last study as an example, it is possible that high levels of church attendance, stricter gun controls, and lower rates of suicide are all products of some underlying variable such as social cohesion. Furthermore, the regional comparisons do not permit conclusions about the behavior of individuals (the ecological fallacy), and in Chapter 7 we suggest some directions for the research needed at the individual level of analysis. Despite the weaknesses of particular studies, however, the research presented in this chapter as a whole, together with the studies reported in Chapter 4 on the relationship between actual firearm ownership and suicide rates, builds a strong case for the thesis that the availability of firearms is powerfully related to their use in suicide.

—6—

Displacement Between Methods

With the jumpers and the drowners, McGee, you don't pick up a pattern. That's because a jumper damned near always makes it the first time, and a drowner is usually almost as successful, about the same rate as hangers. They get cut down maybe as rarely as the drowners get pulled out. So the patterns mostly come from the bleeders and the pill-takers and the shooters. Funny how many people survive a self-shooting. But if they don't destroy a chunk of their brain, they get a chance at a second try. Like the bleeders cut themselves again, and the pill-takers keep trying. It's always patterns. Never change. They pick the way that they want to go and keep after it until they make it. A pill-taker doesn't turn into a jumper, and a drowner won't shoot himself. Like they've got one picture of dying and that's it and there's no other way of going. (John MacDonald, *The Girl in the Plain Brown Wrapper*, 1968, p. 102)

It should be clear from the variety of time series and regional studies presented in this book that the increased availability of a lethal agent—whether guns or carbon monoxide in car exhausts and domestic gas—results in the increased use of that method for suicide. Less certain, however, is whether this increased availability also results in an overall rise in suicide. However, this question needs to be answered unequivocally because of the implications for prevention. There is little point in restricting the availability of a particular lethal agent if the only consequence is that the suicidal person switches, or "displaces," to some other lethal method. This issue is examined here, beginning with some definitions and discussion of methodology.

The Concept of Displacement

As used in this book, the term *displacement* refers to the substitution of one method of suicide for another whose availability has been reduced. We have borrowed the term from the criminological literature, where it refers to the idea that blocking the opportunity for a particular crime simply results in its displacement to some other place or time, another method, or even some other kind of offense (Reppetto, 1976; Gabor, 1978).

Displacement has been seen to pose a particular threat to crime prevention through environmental design (or "situational prevention," as it is termed in Britain). In our view, however, the concept has gained much spurious validity as a result of the predominantly "dispositional bias" of most criminological theory—the tendency to neglect the situational determinants of crime in favor of person-centered variable (see Clarke and Mayhew, 1980).[1] In fact, much evidence exists that situational factors can greatly affect the probability of crime, particularly with respect to impulsive or opportunistic offenses. In addition, recent studies of displacement suggest that its threat has been exaggerated. Numerous examples exist of real gains achieved through situational preventive measures, and there is also evidence that preventive benefits may sometimes spill over beyond the immediate targets of action (Clarke, in press).

Even if a more skeptical attitude is now taken of displacement in the crime prevention field, most common sense views, and indeed the major theories, still regard displacement as a fatal objection to the idea of preventing suicide by restricting access to lethal agents. Suicide is, after all, rarely opportunistic or implusive in the sense that these terms apply to crime, and anyone wishing to die can surely find a method even if his or her preferred route is blocked.

The next chapter examines the validity of these contentions, but in the meantime it is important to arrive at some overall judgment of the extent of displacement resulting from restricted access to lethal agents. Many difficulties are involved in doing this, even if the possibilities for displacement are much more limited for suicide than for crime. First, a large reduction in the use of one method of suicide might be followed by smaller and less visible increases in the use of some, but perhaps not all, other methods. Second, displacement may be only partial, thus also increasing the difficulty of detection. Third, when suicide in general is increasing, which was the case during the period when most of the relevant research was conducted, this rather than displacement may explain an increase in other forms of suicide following a reduction in a particular method. Indeed, the effect of domestic gas detoxification in the Netherlands may well have been masked by a general rise in suicide (Study 2). Fourth, a decrease in

---

[1] This is a general tendency of social science (Jones, 1979), and it may not be surprising that varieties of the displacement criticism have arisen in a number of fields. For example, behavior therapists have had to content with the concept of "symptom substitution," the supposedly inevitable appearance of fresh symptoms of a neurotic disorder following the eradication of earlier ones, advocates of restricting the supply of drugs have had to deal with the "escalation" hypothesis under which people stopped from obtaining "soft" drugs are presumed to turn instead to "harder" drugs, and safety engineers have been forced to consider the concept of "risk homeostasis," under which, for example, the development of safer cars is said to lead to more reckless driving (Wilde, 1986; Orr, 1984). We do not suggest these concepts are without validity, only that their importance may have been exaggerated.

opportunities for one method of suicide might be accompanied by an independent increase in those for a second (as occurred in the United States when detoxification of domestic gas coincided with an increase in the availability of automobiles; Study 3). In these circumstances, it is difficult to establish how much of any increase in the use of the second method is due to displacement. Fifth, when displacement is to a less lethal method, with which death is less frequently the result, it is more difficult to detect because records on attempted suicides are incomplete (Wells, 1981). However, this sort of displacement poses less of a threat to the opportunity-reducing perspective because the net result is still a saving of lives.

A final source of difficulty in studying displacement in the context of suicide is that it refers not just to the behavior or *individuals* who seek some other method when they cannot kill themselves in a particular way, but also to the apparent tendency of *populations* to exploit or develop new forms of suicide in response to a decline in formerly available opportunities. This latter form of displacement may take some time to manifest itself as populations become familiar with the new method. It may be unclear therefore whether the changes taking place are really due to displacement or to some other factor, such as a change in fashion or in the availability of an alternative method. For example, the recent increase in car exhaust poisonings in Britain (Study 4) may be a result of some delayed displacement as the result of the detoxification of domestic gas, but it is just as likely to have resulted from increased availability of cars (and possibly also garages) and from increased familiarity with and greater acceptance of the method. These changes may have occurred even without detoxification of domestic gas.

Evidence from the Present Studies

Acknowledging the difficulties of studying displacement, what conclusions can we derive from our own and others' research?

To begin with guns, the evidence from the regional studies of firearm availability is somewhat mixed. When the accidental death rate from guns and the percentage of homicides using guns were used as indices of firearm availability in each state (Study 6), it was found that displacement to firearm use may have occurred. Similar findings were produced by Study 8 based on the nine major regions of the United States and on the Australian states. In contrast, gun magazine subscriptions used as an index of firearm availability were found to be associated with both the firearm suicide rate and the total suicide rate, suggesting that additional firearms create additonal suicides (Study 7). A similar result was obtained in the study of the strictness of handgun control laws in the United States (Study 10), which found that states with stricter handgun control laws had lower firearm suicide rates and lower overall suicide rates. Suicide rates by poisons and hanging/

strangulation were not related to firearm availability, suggesting that switching does not occur to any great extent.

The most relevant result from the time-series analysis of gun ownership in the United States (Study 9) was that as the firearm suicide rate increased the suicide rate by all other methods decreased. This suggests that some of those who might have used other methods for suicide did switch to firearms. However, the increase in the firearm suicide rate from 1959 to 1984 was 2.5 per 100,000 per year while the drop in suicide rate by all other methods was only 0.7. This is consistent with the idea that the increased availability of handguns created *additional* suicides rather than merely changing the methods people chose for killing themselves.

To summarize, two studies of firearms (7, 10) suggest that increased availability of guns creates additional suicides, two do not (6, 8), and the third (9) suggests that some but not complete displacement occurs. Some of the ambiguity in these results may be a result of poor measurement of gun ownership.

Turning to the studies on car exhaust, a regional analysis of the states in the United States (Study 4) indicated that the more cars per capita in a state, the higher the suicide rate by car exhaust while the suicide rate by all other methods remained unrelated to the extent of car ownership. This suggests that switching methods for suicide did not take place, though this conclusion must be treated with caution since suicide by car exhaust is not a common method in the United States. The time-series study of the effect of emission controls in the United States (Study 5) showed that these did halt the rising suicide rate by car exhaust, but no conclusions could be reached about displacement to other methods.

The clearest findings related to displacement were produced by Study 1 on the detoxification of domestic gas in England and Wales. Detoxification resulted in a dramatic decrease in domestic gas suicides without a corresponding increase in the suicide rate by other methods. In this case the reduced opportunity to commit suicide saved thousands of lives. Study 5 suggests, however, that a small amount of delayed displacement may have occurred subsequently, in the form of increased use of car exhaust suicides.

The results of the studies of gas detoxification in Scotland and the Netherlands (Study 2) and in the United States (Study 3) were more suggestive of displacement, though we believe alternative explanations are available in these other cases. In Scotland and in the Netherlands, detoxification of domestic gas took place during a period of rising suicide rates, which might have obscured any decrease in the suicide rate resulting from the reduced toxicity of domestic gas. In the United States, detoxification coincided largely with a period just after World War II when cars were becoming much more available and consequently opportunities for suicide using exhaust gas were greatly increased.

Availability of Drugs

Although we ourselves have conducted to research on the availability of drugs, several studies permit comment on the issue of displacement.[2] Oliver and Hetzel (1972, 1973) examined the impact in Australia of the July 1967 imposition of restrictions on sedative prescriptions (mainly for barbiturates, but later extended to other hypnotics) as a result of rising concern over the use of these drugs in self-poisoning. Their results (reproduced in the following table) show a close relationship between the number of sedative tablets issued and numbers of drug suicides:

	Drug suicides	Other suicides	Tablets issued (100 millions)
1961	276	973	2.74
1962	395	1074	3.82
1963	610	1108	4.57
1964	601	1019	5.06
1965	686	999	5.48
1966	655	969	5.64
1967	719	1059	5.03
1968	548	979	4.80
1969	539	963	4.65
1970	501	1050	4.20

More important, these figures show no evidence of displacement *away* from other methods as sedative-related suicides increased in frequency up to 1967 and no displacement *to* other methods after controls were imposed on prescribing.

A closely similar pattern of results was demonstrated by Whitlock (1975) in his study of barbiturate overdoses in Brisbane (suicides increased in line with increased availability of these drugs and declined following prescription

---

[2] One interesting study that, unfortunately, does not permit any comment on displacement is that by Clarke (1985). He reports that in 1909 an act of Parliament in Great Britain restricted the sale of opiates by labeling drugs with more than 1 percent of morphine as "poisons," which required purchasers to register with the pharmacist and sign for the drug. A later act, in 1916, lowered the critical concentration to 0.75 percent morphine, and an act of 1921 required a prescription for the first time if the concentration of morphine was over 0.2 percent. In 1852 to 1856, completed suicides by opiates constituted 2.7 percent of all suicides, in 1901 to 1905 2.1 percent, and in 1921 to 1925 only 0.2 percent. Similarly, in 1852 to 1856 completed suicide by opiates constituted 25.9 percent of all suicides by poison, in 1901 to 1905, 12.2, and in 1921 to 1925 only 2.1 percent. However, the number of suicides by opiates was so small that elimination of their availability would have had little impact on the overall suicide rate.

controls, with no evidence of any displacement). It therefore appears firmly established that restrictions on the prescribing of sedatives in Australia reduced the number of drug suicides without increasing suicides by other methods.

In Japan, Yamasawa et al. (1980) noted (and illustrated with graphs) that in 1956 for the first time prescriptions were required for hypnotic drugs. The result was a decrease in the suicide rate by drugs and chemicals, with no parallel increase in the use of agricultural chemicals or cyanide salts.

In Scotland, McMurray et al. (1987) have shown, with data from a district poisons unit for 1971 through 1985, that the rise and fall of admissions for deliberate self-poisoning paralleled the availability of barbiturates. For England and Wales, Brewer and Farmer (1985) have argued that drug suicides declined from 1977 to 1983 in company with a reduced number of prescriptions for hypnotics and tranquilizers. They further pointed out that, because the overall rate of suicide fell in England and Wales after 1981, no displacement to other methods of suicide occurred.

In another British study, Henry (1988) has published data for 1974 through 1984 showing the "fatal toxicity indices" (FTIs) for the major antidepressants in use during the period. FTIs are the number of recorded death due to overdoses per million prescriptions written for each drug. The results (summarized in Table 6.1) show very large differences in FTIs between the various drugs, with the more recent antidepressants generally being much safer. Since there is no evidence that patients prescribed a particular drug are more likely to attempt suicide than patients prescribed an alternative, these differences are likely to be a result of differences in the toxicity of the drugs. Had some depressed patients been prescribed less toxic drugs, they may not have died. Henry concludes: "If the newer drugs have as good a record of clinical effectiveness combined with their apparent lower potential to cause fatal poisoning when taken in overdose, serious consideration should be given to preferentially prescribing the newer drugs, especially in situations where suicidal overdose is a possibility" (p. 51).

These examples, from different countries and involving different drugs, show that the availability of a particular chemical is powerfully related to its use in suicide. Prescribing the more toxic antidepressants results in more suicides from overdoses, and when restrictions on prescribing (principally of sedatives) have been introduced their use for suicide has declined. Moreover, results from several of the studies suggest that the declining use of a drugs for suicide is not accompanied by displacement to other methods. It is unlikely that any alternative explanatory factor could be advanced to account for the results. For example, it is unlikely that improvements in emergency medical treatment occurred in 1967 in Australia (as was suggested by Gibbs and Arnold, 1972) *and* in 1956 in Japan. Clearly no such explanation could account for the large differences in the risk of fatal overdose between antidepressants in Great Britain.

Table 6.1. Deaths from overdoses of antidepressants per million prescriptions Great Britain, 1974–1984.

Drug	Number of deaths	Deaths per million prescriptions
	Tricylic antidepressants	
Dibenzepin	4	157.5[b]
Desipramine	13	80.2[b]
Dothiepin	533	50.0[a]
Amitriptyline	1181	46.5[a]
Nortriptyline	57	39.2NS
Doxepin	102	31.3NS
Imipramine	278	28.4[a]
Trimipramine	155	27.6[b]
Opipramol	2	21.8NS
Clomipramine	51	11.1[a]
Protriptyline	6	10.3[b]
Iprindole	2	7.8[b]
	Monoamine oxidase inhibitors	
Tranylcypromine	15	58.1NS
Phenylzine	24	22.8[c]
Isocarboxazid	3	12.8[c]
Iproniazid	0	0.0NS
	Antidepressants introduced after 1973	
Maprotiline	83	77.0	37.6NS
Trazodone	6	15.0	13.6[c]
Viloxazine	2	7.4	9.4[c]
Butriptyline	1	4.7	7.5NS
Mianserin	30	187.0	5.6[a]
Nomifensine	3	42.0	2.5[a]
Lofepramine	0	3.7	0.0NS

[a] $P < 0.001$ from means for all antidepressants (2551 deaths, 34.9 per million prescriptions).
[b] $P < 0.01$
[c] $P < 0.05$
NS = not significantly different from the mean of 34.9 per million.
Source: Henry (1988).

Conclusions

In an analysis of suicide deaths in England and Wales for the hundred years from 1876 to 1975, Farmer (1979) found that those by domestic gas poisoning for the whole period and those by other poisonings in the last 25 years varied independently of the other methods. That these methods did not increase as others decreased (or vice versa) led Farmer to suggest that "the factors influencing suicide mortality by one method may differ from those influencng mortality by another method, in part at least" (p. 779). He went on to argue that "this hypothesis is certainly an attractive one in the case of suicidal domestic gas poisonings, since their numbers correlate with gas supply. Furthermore the change in the numbers of poisonings by solid and liquid substance is consistent with the increase in the supply of drugs since the second war" (p. 779).

If one accepts Farmer's explanation for his results, as we do, one would not expect much displacement between methods of suicide following changes in availability. This is consistent with the evidence from our own studies of suicide by guns and domestic or exhaust gases, as well as from studies of self-poisoning in Australia, Britain, and Japan. This suggests that the changed availability of a method for suicide affects not only its use for suicide but also the overall rate of suicide, even when some displacement occurs. In the case of detoxification of domestic gas in England and Wales, the effect on the overall suicide rate was dramatic.

How much displacement is to be expected, and under what conditions, is not well understood. We believe that little progress will be made by simply repeating the kind of time-series and regional studies that we have undertaken; a fresh research approach is needed.

In the next chapter we make some suggestions concerning the form that this should take, but a reorientation of causal theory is also needed. The prevailing sociological and psychological theories of suicide—of which the former, following Durkheim, locate the causes of suicide in social disintegration, and the latter, deriving from the psychoanalytic school, see suicide as resulting from personal disturbance and depression—do not attach much importance to the availability of a lethal agent. Nor would either have predicted the magnitude of the fall in suicide witnessed in England and Wales following gas detoxification. Indeed, both theoretical positions assume that a "genuinely" suicidal person will always find a method, and displacement is generally to be expected.

If, as we propose in the final chapter, more theoretical importance were attached to the thought and decision processes that underlie and sustain each act of suicide, it would be much easier to see that opportunity can play an important part in the final act and that displacement may not be inevitable.

Thus, the fact that few people in England and Wales killed themselves in some other way when deprived of toxic gas is perhaps explained by the very real advantages of this means of death. Not only was it highly lethal, but it was painless, clean, easy, and required relatively little courage or preparation. Unable to identify an equally acceptable alternative, most of the individuals concerned seem to have abandoned the idea or, perhaps, tried but failed to kill themselves with some less lethal method. It would not be surprising, however, if reduced availability of a method with fewer advantages than domestic gas were followed by more displacement. Nor would it be surprising if *increases* in availability were less likely to result in displacement than *decreases*, since it may take longer to recognize the existence of new opportunities than discover that old ones have been foreclosed.

Rather than regard suicide as an essentially homogeneous category of behavior, it may therefore be more profitable to treat it as a collection of separate but related behaviors distinguished by the method and populations involved. The degree of displacement between different methods would therefore be much less than is commonly thought. There may also be "specialists" in less lethal methods such as wrist-slashing or overdosing. Moreover, as Farmer and Rohde (1980) argue, national and local variations in methods used resulting from differential opportunities for suicide may reflect differences in the *incidence* of suicide as much as in the forms it takes.

Finally, we return to a point made earlier in this chapter about the dual nature of the concept of displacement: it refers both to the behavior of individuals who seek an alternative when a preferred route to suicide is blocked and to the behavior of populations in exploiting or developing replacements for a formerly available method. In discussions of the potential benefits of controlling lethal agents, these two aspects of displacement tend to become confused. Frequently, it is assumed that nothing is to be gained by opportunity-reducing methods if the only result is that in a few years some other method takes its place. However, this overlooks the fact that many people, if prevented from suicide at a particular time, find other solutions to their difficulties and may never kill themselves. Thus, even if in the longer term a new method begins to replace one that has been removed (as may have occurred in Britain, where car exhaust suicides have increased in popularity since domestic gas detoxification), many thousands of lives might have been saved in the interim.

7

Explaining Choice of Method

Richard had decided somehow, sometime ago, that if he ever felt like killing himself, he would use car exhaust. Certainly, he hadn't the temperament to cut his wrists. He had even measured the diameter of the exhaust pipe on his car. His thoughts turned to where he could buy some rubber tubing.... About a mile down the road he noticed a hardware store open. He parked and went in, nervously. He walked up and down the aisles looking for likely tubing. He found the water hoses but they were too narrow to fit over the exhaust pipe.... He hesitated, but approached an assistant. "How much do you want sir?" "Ten feet. No, make it two ten feet pieces." Would that be enough? Probably. How was he going to fit it over the exhaust pipes? He needed some clamps. He found them just as the assistant returned, carrying two long poles. He noted Richard's alarm. "It's the freezing weather, sir. They harden up. They'll get flexible when they're warm.".... Richard carried them out and opened the trunk of his car. He put them in crosswise, but they extended too far to fit into the trunk completely. They resisted. He would get one bent into the trunk but, when he tackled the second, the first one would spring out. On the fourth try, the trunk closed. "Damn the blasted tubes." (Taken from an account of a client of one of the authors who never did attempt suicide.)

In the previous chapter we reviewed evidence from our own and other research regarding displacement following changes in the availability of a lethal agent. A number of studies, particularly of firearms, suggest that some switching between methods takes place as a result of changes in availability. Other studies, including some of guns but more especially those concerned with domestic gas and sedatives and antidepressants, suggest that displacement is, at best, only partial. The most fully documented case, that of detoxification of domestic gas in England and Wales, found very little displacement, possibly because this method has particular advantages. It is painless, easy, clean, requires little preparation, and is highly lethal. No other method may offer this combination of advantages and thus afford a realistic alternative for many would-be suicides.

Although most theorists would resist the idea that the properties of a method may significantly influence the decision to commit suicide, it has been recognized since Durkheim (1897) that psychological and cultural factors influence choice of method. This observation received little careful attention, however, until the early 1960s (Hirsh, 1960; Dublin, 1963). Dublin distinguished three determining factors in choice of method: (1) availability or accessibility, (2) suggestion or infectiousness, and (3) personal and symbolic factors. With slight modifications, this classification provides a convenient starting point for the following discussion.

Availability and Accessibility

A common criticism of the proposal to reduce opportunities for suicide is that the most "available" methods are, in fact, not the ones most frequently used. The point is expressed by Marks and Abernathy (1974) as follows:

What are the most physically available methods in the United States for an individual to kill himself? Submersion? Cutting? Hanging? Burning? Jumping from a high place? Jumping in front of a speeding motor vehicle? Surely these are some of the most physically available methods for a person who wants to kill himself; however, these available methods are not used most frequently. Thus any explanation of differential methods of suicide... cannot be based solely on the logic of the physical presence (availability) of any given method for self-destruction" (p. 7).

Combining the notion of accessibility with availability makes it easier to deal with this criticism, however, because it permits the influence of geography to be accommodated in explaining choice of method as well as of differences in the suicidal person's physical and mental capacities. For example, a city worker with an office in a tall building may have much greater access to jumping as a method of suicide than his suburban neighbor who works locally. Country dwellers may find it easier to find a private place to hang themselves (for example, a secluded tree) than people living in towns and cities. People with cars might more easily get to places where they could drown or throw themselves from a height. Anyone with a bit of technical competence is in a better position to use exhaust gas than someone without. Those who cannot swim can more easily drown themselves. Police have greater access to guns for suicide (Friedman, 1967) and chemists to poisons (Li, 1969). And we have suggested (in Study 2) that gas suicide may have been less common in the Netherlands because the design of gas fires and cookers made them difficult to use for that purpose.

These and other practical aspects of availability and accessibility may be important in causation since, quite early in the process of contemplating suicide, most people have to think hard about what method to use. Failure to identify a suitable method or to resolve the practical difficulties involved could result in the idea of suicide being abandoned.

Suggestion and Symbolism

Phillips (1974) has documented the possibility that publicity following suicides may increase the rate of suicide and that there are fashions in the methods used. He found that front-page news stories on suicide were followed by an increase in the number of suicides in the following month and, in a more recent study (Phillips and Carstensen, 1988), found a similar effect following television news reports of suicides. Many examples of suggestion have also been found in the literature, in both historical accounts of imitation or mass suicide and case histories of individuals.[1]

One of the most famous of these examples is the wave of suicides in the late eighteenth century triggered by Goethe's romantic novel, *The Sorrows of Young Werther*, about a lovesick youth who kills himself with his successful rival's pistol. Copies of the book were found on the bodies of so many suicides that a Protestant pastor denounced Goethe as a murderer, sale of the book was banned in Leipzig, and the clergy in Milan bought up the entire printing of the Italian edition.

A more recent and better documented example of the power of suggestion and symbolism is to be found in the story of Mount Mihara in Japan, which became a suicide shrine in the early 1930s (Ellis and Allen, 1961). Until that time, Mount Mihara, which is on an island some 60 miles from Tokyo, attracted only a few tourists who went to see the sulfur clouds from its volcano. However, in January 1933, a pupil from an exclusive girls' school in Tokyo jumped into the crater, only to be followed a month later by another girl from the same school.

The deaths attracted enormous publicity, and the legend took hold that those who jumped were instantly cremated and their souls sent heavenward in a plume of smoke. Crowds of sightseers flocked to the island and on one Sunday in April, 6 of these sightseers plunged into the crater while another 25 had to be forcibly restrained. The crowds of the curious could soon almost rely on seeing a suicide each day, and by the end of 1933, 133 known suicides had occurred and many more were suspected.

Despite strenuous policing efforts (by the end of 1934 the police had forcibly prevented more than 1200 people from jumping into the volcano), the problem continued, with 619 death in 1936 alone. A fence was built which, along with some other preventive steps, reduced the lure of the mountain. Suicides did not cease, however, until 1955 when a badly injured young couple who had leaped like so many before was rescued from 500 yards deep in the crater. Their rescue destroyed the myth of instant cremation that seemed to have exerted so poweful a fascination on so many people.

A less remarkable series of events, but one that recently caused considerable consternation in the northeastern United States, originated in a

---

[1] A recent example of the influence of availability and symbolism of a weapon is provided by White-Bowden (1985), who described the case of her son, Jodie, who shot himself at home at the age of 17 following problems at school and rejection by a girl friend. A few years previously the boy's father had also shot himself in the same house when unable to face the finality of divorce from his wife. The fact that a gun was still available in the house not only made it easier for the boy to follow his father's example but also to identify with his father's psychological state.

well-publicized case of suicide by four teenagers in Bergenfield, New Jersey. The facts are as follows.[2] At 6:30 a.m. on March 12, 1987, four teenagers were found dead in a car with the engine running, parked in a 13-car garage of an apartment complex in Bergenfield (a community of 25,000 people about 10 miles from the George Washington Bridge which links New Jersey to Manhattan). A suicide note signed by all four said that they wanted to be buried together. The time of death was estimated at between 4 and 5:30 a.m.

The four belonged to a group of teenagers who were known as the burn-outs. In the previous summer, four of the group had died in accidents, including one who fell from the Pallisade Cliffs to his death while walking with one of the victims in the car.

In the following week several teenage suicides by car exhaust were reported in other cities, including one by a youth in Clifton, New Jersey, on March 17. Then in Bergenfield, on March 18 at just after 4 a.m., two teenagers, a boy and a girl, were found by the police in a car in the *same* garage used the previous week by the four suicides. The boy had turned off the engine when he heard the police officer arrive.

The two teenagers knew the four who had died the previous week. The girl had made three suicide attempts in recent years and had received psychiatric treatment. The day before her suicide attempt, her sister had told the police that she was suicidal, and she had been taken to see a psychiatrist.

Because of the anxiety in Bergenfield in the days following the first four suicides, suicide crisis hotlines had been set up, and the police were checking the garage every hour in which the four had died. It was this precaution that saved the two teenagers, for they had only one hour to commit suicide in the garage before it was checked again. After this second use of the garage to attempt suicide, the police removed the door.

The best documented case study of suggestion and symbolism was done by Seiden and Spence (1983–84) on suicide from the Golden Gate and Bay Bridges which, respectively, link San Francisco with the counties of northern California and the cities on the East Bay. During the approximately 40 years from their opening in 1937, nearly 800 suicides were confirmed at these locations. However, suicides from the Golden Gate Bridge outnumbered those from the Bay Bridge by more than five to one (671:121).

Seiden and Spence's study investigates the reasons for this difference in risk between the two bridges, which are similar in many other respects: they were opened within a few months of each other, they are in close proximity of each other, and they are of approximately the same height (200 feet above the water). Certain other factors might have been expected to favor the Bay

---

[2] Details are taken from editions of the *New York Times*, March 1987.

Bridge as a suicide site: it is about eight times as long and carries about twice as much traffic (about 194,000 vehicles per day compared with 98,000 for the Golden Gate Bridge). One important difference favoring the Golden Gate Bridge, however, is that it is accessible to pedestrians, whereas the Bay Bridge is open only to vehicles. Of 555 suicides from the Golden Gate Bridge studied by Seiden and Spence, 230 had been on foot, whereas this was the case for only 5 out of 112 suicides from the Bay Bridge. Nevertheless, still three times as many suicides from the Golden Gate drove onto the bridge in cars, suggesting other factors were at work than accessibility.

This conclusion is reinforced by the fact that of East Bay residents (served primarily by the Bay Bridge) who used a car to get to their suicide site, as many jumped from the Golden Gate (58) as from the Bay Bridge (57). Indeed, about half of the 58 who used the Golden Gate would have to have crossed the Bay Bridge to get there. In additon, as Seiden and Spence observe: "There are even a few people from outside the State of California who travel to San Francisco to jump off the Golden Gate bridge. The Bay bridge, however, has never had a jumper who was not a resident of the State of California" (p. 207). Part of the explanation for this may be that Golden Gate suicides often receive front page coverage while those from the Bay Bridge rarely do.

Seiden and Spence see these facts as evidence of the "symbolically determined and romanticized attractiveness of the Golden Gate Bridge vis-a-vis the Bay Bridge" and of "a commonly held attitude that often romanticizes suicides from the Golden Gate in such terms as 'aesthetically pleasing' and 'beautiful' while regarding Bay Bridge suicides as 'tacky' and 'declasse'" (p. 207). In support, they quote Rosen's (1975) interviews with a handful of Golden Gate suicide survivors, as a result of which he characterized the bridge as "suicide shrine" with unique meaning to the jumpers—a meaning associated with death, grace, and beauty.

Personal Requirements and Cultural Norms

All of us fear death, but some forms of death are more terrifying than others. Thus, most of us dread a long terminal illness with severe pain and progressive loss of functions. Indeed, quality of death may be as meaningful a concept to most people as quality of life. However, the desiderata of death, in particular of a suicidal death, depends on personal circumstances. Most suicidal individuals are concerned about the physical pain involved and many, particularly women (Marks, 1977), about the damage to their faces and bodies. Some individuals, for religious reasons or to safeguard insurance payments for their relatives, may want to conceal the suicidal nature of their deaths while others, particularly those who commit suicide in a public way such as by jumping under a subway train (Guggenheim and Weisman, 1972), may wish the opposite. Punishing people they consider responsible for their plight may be important in some cases, whereas others may wish to cause the minimum of distress.

All of these considerations are likely to influence the choice of method though they have not been much studied. Dublin's (1963) own work concentrated mainly on the concept of lethality of intent. For example, he sought to explain the greater use of firearms by males primarily on the grounds that men who attempt suicide have more lethal intent than women whose suicide attempts are more often manipulative. For the manipulative or ambivalent, slower methods are usually preferred since these might allow either a last minute change of mind or fate to have a hand, for example, through the chance intervention of a lover or friend.

Some dangers of circular reasoning implicit in the concept of lethality of intent (any method used in a completed suicide is "lethal") were discussed by Marks and Abernathy (1974), who argued that men's greater use of firearms reflects, instead, their greater familiarity with and acceptance of guns. These investigators also put forward the same reason for the generally greater use of guns in suicide in the southern states (Marks and Stokes, 1976). Indeed, the concept of differential socialization has wider relevance than merely for the use of guns. For example, Durkheim observed that Englishmen rarely hang themselves, perhaps because hanging is the traditional punishment in England for traitors and murderers. We have suggested (Study 5) that car exhaust suicides might be more common in the United States because of the salience of the car in everyday life. And as Noomen (1975) has observed in commenting on the high incidence of suicide by drowning in Holland; "The Dutchman knows about death, because he knows about the water" (p. 168).

Choice Structuring Properties of Methods of Suicide

Marks and Abernathy (1974) identify five variables that would help to explain an individual's preference for a particular method of self-destruction: its physical availability, the actor's knowledge of the method, his familiarity with the method, his personal or social accessibility to the method, and his evaluation of the method. With a little thought, and drawing on the work of others discussed previously, their list can be considerably extended, and we offer 20 "choice structuring properties" (Cornish and Clarke, 1989) we believe attach in various degrees to the method of suicide chosen (poisoning, cutting, suffocation and hanging, drowning, electrocution, shooting, jumping, etc.):

1. Availability (e.g., own a car?)
2. Familiarity with the method (e.g., car exhaust gases)
3. Technical skills needed (hanging, gasing)
4. Planning necessary (buy a gun, save up drugs)
5. Likely pain (cutting wrists)

6. "Courage" needed (high building, train)
7. Consequences of failure (disability, publicity)
8. Disfigurement after death (hanging versus overdose)
9. Danger/inconvenience to others (car crash, subway leap)
10. Messiness/bloodiness (wrist cutting)
11. Discovery of body (by loved ones or strangers)
12. "Contamination" of nest (i.e., avoid home)
13. Scope for concealing or publicizing death—shame, insurance (car-crash, drowning, subway leap)
14. Certainty of death (perceived/actual)
15. Time taken to die while conscious (poisons, wrist cutting)
16. Scope for second thoughts (swim back to shore, switch off gas)
17. Chances of intervention ("fate," estranged lover)
18. Symbolism (cleansing by fire, seppuku)
19. Masculine/feminine (e.g., guns)
20. Dramatic impact (lover's leap versus overdose)

These properties are largely self-explanatory and should require no further illustration. Their relative importance is unknown, however, and other significant properties may have been omitted. Further, some of the properties are related in practice (for example, most bloody methods may need courage) and they can be conceptually linked under more general dimensions of opportunities (1–4 in the list), costs (5–13) and (14–20) of the various methods. Finally, some of the costs and benefits have both positive and negative valences, depending on the motivation of the individual concerned; for example, one individual may wish to spare relations the shock of discovering the body whereas someone else may deliberately inflict this them.

We believe that closer investigation of the reasons for choosing particular methods could help in predicting the likelihood and extent of displacement following changes in the availability of methods. In the case of completed suicides, it may not be possible to do more than infer reasons for choice on the basis of the actions completed. An alternative source of data would be systematic questioning of samples of people, either groups of the suicidally inclined or the general population, to discover what people know about the various methods and how they evaluate them.

Little research has been conducted along these lines, although a study by Marks (1977) illustrates the approach. He questioned a sample of 642 college students about their preferences for method in an effort to understand differences in the choice of methods between men and women. Significant differences were found between the two groups in their evaluations of six of nine methods. Women associated painlessness and efficiency with drugs and poison, whereas men associated masculinity, efficiency, and knowledgeness of method with firearms. This research has influenced the design of the two studies reported nexts, which further illustrate the more detailed work that needs to be undertaken.

Perception of Different Methods
Study 13

Students' perceptions of two relatively common methods of suicide, shooting and overdosing, were compared in this study. A questionnaire was given to 29 male and 43 female undergraduates, 18 to 22 years old, who completed it anonymously. The students were asked to state their preference for guns or an overdose of pills as a method of suicide. They then rated each method of suicide on seven-point rating scales for the following 10 properties, which were judged to be particularly important for the two methods: quick–slow, painful–painless, difficult–easy, irreversible–reversible, good–bad, courageous–cowardly, dramatic–banal, masculine–feminine, messy–tidy, and impulsive–planned.

The respondents viewed suicide by guns and by overdose of pills as different on 9 of the 10 properties (two-tailed $p < .01$ or better for all 9). Suicide by guns was seen as quick (mean score 1.50 on a scale of 1–7), painful (3.26), difficult (3.15), irreversible (1.93), dramatic (2.56), masculine (2.89), and messy (1.54) and as moderately courageous (4.51) and impulsive (4.10). In contrast, an overdose of pills was seen as slow (mean score 5.56), painless (5.47), easy (5.12), cowardly (5.49), feminine (5.35), tidy (6.10), and planned (5.06) and as moderately reversible (4.81) and banal (4.31). (Good–bad ratings did not differentiate the methods.)

The males and females did not differ in their rating of guns as a method for suicide on any of the 10 scales and differed on only one of their ratings of on overdose of pills. (The females saw pills as a little more painless than the males, did—means 5.79 and 5.26, respectively, $F(1,68) = 4.11$, $p = 0.05$).

Students who chose guns ($n = 19$) differed from students who chose an overdose of pills ($n = 53$) in their perception of guns as a method for suicide on only one scale. Those students who chose guns saw them as a little quicker than those who chose an overdose of pills (means scores 1.05 and 1.66, respectively, $F(1,68) = 4.62$, $p = 0.04$).

Students who chose an overdose of pills ($n = 53$) differed from those students who chose guns ($n = 19$) in their perception of an overdose of pills on four scales. They saw pills as less slow (mean scores 5.28 and 6.32, $F(1,68) = 5.53$, $p = 0.02$), more painless (means 5.72 and 4.79, $F(1,68) = 6.71$, $p = 0.01$), less planned (means 4.79 and 5.79, $F(1,68) = 4.51$, $p = 0.04$), and less bad (means 4.79 and 5.95, $F(1,68) = 6.46$, $p = 0.01$).

Thus, the methods of suicide considered in this study (guns and pills) were perceived very differently, and these perceptions were not greatly affected by the sex of the respondent or by the method that the respondent would choose for suicide.

Reasons for Choice of Method
Study 14

Although the previous study showed that different methods of suicide are perceived very differently, further research is needed to explore (1) why one method of suicide is preferred over another, and (2) under what conditions people would switch methods if their preferred method were not available. The present study represents a preliminary investigation of the first of these questions by asking an undergraduate population which method it would choose for suicide and why.

A questionnaire given to 429 students, aged 18 to 22 enrolled in college courses asked: (1) which method they would choose for suicide, (2) whether they chose that method because it is quick, painless, does not disfigure, or is easily available (answered on a five-point rating scale from "not at all" to "definitely"), and (3) how much seven consequences of death concerned them (answered on a five-point rating scale from "doesn't concern me much at all" to "concerns me a lot"). The seven consequences were as follows:

1. I could no longer have any experiences.
2. I am uncertain as to what might happen to me if there is a life after death.
3. I am afraid of what might happen to my body after death,
4. I could no longer care for my dependents.
5. My death would cause grief to my relatives and friends.
6. All my plans and projects would come to an end.
7. The process of dying might be painful.

As expected, there were sex differences in the choice of method. Among the most common methods, females chose an overdose of medication more than males, with a ratio of 1.57:1, guns far less often, with a ratio of 0.35, and carbon monoxide/car exhaust equally often, with a ratio of 1.04 (chi-square $= 43.62$, df $= 2$, $p < 0.001$).

Overall, the females rated painlessness, less disfigurement, and availability as more important reasons for choosing a method for suicide than did the males and availability as less important (see Table 7.1). For those students who chose an overdose of medication (the most common method chosen), females rated the painlessness and availability as more important reasons than did the males (see Table 7.1).

Those who chose guns (rather than an overdose or carbon monoxide) rated quickness as significantly more relevant to their choice ($F = 28.89$, df $= 2/287$, $p < 0.001$) and the disfigurement as less important ($F = 33.92$, df $= 2/287$, $p < 0.001$) but did not differ in their ratings of the importance of pain and availability ($F = 2.09$ and 2.24, respectively).

To check the importance of lack of disfigurement, the concern for "I am afraid of what might happen to my body after death" was examined. Those

Table 7.1. Sex differences in reasons for choosing a particular method for suicide.

| | Females | | Males | | | |
	Mean	SD	Mean	SD	t	p
All subjects						
Quick	3.9	(1.1)	3.8	(1.3)	0.35	ns
Painless	4.5	(0.9)	4.0	(1.3)	4.17	< 0.001
Not disfiguring	3.7	(1.4)	2.8	(1.6)	5.61	< 0.001
Available	4.0	(1.1)	3.6	(1.4)	3.33	= 0.001
n	191		237			
Those choosing overdoses						
Quick	3.7	(1.1)	3.4	(1.2)	1.91	ns
Painless	4.6	(0.7)	4.2	(1.2)	2.53	= 0.01
Not disfiguring	3.8	(1.4)	3.6	(1.4)	1.30	ns
Available	4.1	(1.1)	3.7	(1.3)	2.07	= 0.04
n	116		74			

who chose guns had significantly less concern about this than those who chose overdoses and carbon monoxide, and males had less concern than females. (None of the other six consequences of death were significantly differentiated among those choosing different methods of suicide.)

The results of this study of college students showed that the quickness, painfulness, degree of disfigurement, and availability of methods for suicide do play a role in the hypothetical choice of method for suicide. In particular, females are more concerned about the appearance of their body after death, as are those who choose overdose and carbon monoxide. Also females are more likely to choose overdoses than males.

This suggests that making lethal medications less easily available may indeed lower the overall suicide rate, since people for whom disfigurement is a concern may well not switch to a more disfiguring method of suicide. Similarly, those who choose guns appear to want a quick death and may not switch to a slower and perhaps less certain method.

Conclusions

In the previous chapter we suggested that a fuller understanding of displacement requires a reorientation of theory to give more weight to the thinking and decision-making processes involved in suicide. In this chapter we have advocated, specifically, studying the choice-structuring properties of different methods of suicide by questioning samples of both the at-risk and the general population. Two illustrative studies of the approach were presented showing that undergraduates perceive large differences in the choice-structuring properties of a variety of methods.

More detailed studies are now required, with different populations, of the behavioral implications of these perceptions. The studies need to be extended to depressed presuicidal people as well as to those who have just attempted suicide (both first-time attempters and repeaters). Other ways of eliciting the information need to be explored. The studies reported in this chapter used a modified Semantic Differential technique in which subjects were provided with dimensions on which to rate the methods. More revealing information might result from the use of Repertory Grid techniques (Kelly, 1955) in which the subjects supply their own dimensions.

As mentioned previously, use of a particular method for suicide could increase quite independently of a reduction in the use of another method, through imitation or simply as result of changes in fashion. There may also be a general tendency for populations to exploit or develop novel methods of committing suicide—what might be called "innovation." Investigation of these possibilities, as well as of displacement, may be assisted by further analysis of choice-structuring properties. Research of this kind demands the monitoring of public knowledge about different methods of suicide, how knowledge of new methods is spread, and how different populations evaluate choice-structuring properties.

—8—

Implications for Theory
and Prevention

The evidence presented in previous chapters suggests that the increased availability of a lethal agent increases its use for suicide and, depending on the particular method, may increase the overall suicide rate, creating new suicides rather than merely causing potential suicides to switch methods. Conversely, a decline in the availability of lethal agent leads not only to a fall in the use of that method, but possibly also to a decrease in the overall rate of suicide. Correlational studies of the kind we have reported have well-known limitations for causal analysis, but three aspects of the present set of studies provide powerful support for these propositions:

1. the studies involve a variety of lethal agents,
2. for some of the methods of suicide we have presented time-series *and* regional studies, and
3. the research has used data from a number of different countries.

In this final chapter we draw out the implications of these findings for theory and prevention. We develop the outlines of a "decision" theory of suicide that focuses on the suicidal person's thought processes and decision making, and we discuss a public health approach to prevention; the first and most important component of this approach is greater attention to restricting the availability of lethal agents, such as handguns, poisons, and toxic car exhausts. A supplementary component relates to reducing the acceptability of suicide as a solution to life's problems. We begin by outlining the implications for theory.

A Decision Theory of Suicide

The research described in this volume has important implications for our understanding of suicide. Hitherto, it was easy to think of suicide as a desperate act, committed by seriously dysfunctional people at their wits' end. It seems unlikely that these people would be deterred by having to wait several days for a permit to buy a handgun or several weeks to acquire a lethal quantity of antidepressants.

That availability of lethal agents does influence suicidal behavior suggests, however, that the act of taking one's life is in large measure also a product of situational factors. This is consistent with the crisis model of suicide intervention, which argues that the suicidal crisis is usually temporary and intervention may be needed only to get the suicidal person through a bad night or couple of days.

The effect of situational influences is most easily understood through a theory that focuses on the mental processes underlying and sustaining each act of suicide. These include how an individual predicament becomes defined as hopeless, accompanying feelings of depression, the manner in which solutions are sought and evaluated, how suicide first comes to be entertained, and how plans are made and put into effect. Such a formulation gives considerable importance to the choice-structuring properties of different methods discussed in Chapter 7 and how these are evaluated by those contemplating suicide.

The judgment that life is no longer worth living, the decision to end it, and the choice of method may be interactive rather than sequential. For example, despairing or depressed individuals for whom suicide is prohibited on religious grounds may gradually redefine their situations or find other solutions. Others may support their plan for suicide with thoughts about people who have found it the only way out, and may only give up the idea when they cannot find an acceptable method. Those who do identify a method may go on to develop realistic plans, including a detailed scenario of the place and the time of their deaths. As suggested by the contents of some suicide notes (see, Stengel, 1964), they may carefully plan their funerals and the disposal of their belongings. Elaborate fantasies about the effect of their deaths on others may also be constructed. This mental preparation helps reinforce feelings of hopelessness and the belief that there is no other way out.

While elements of such a theory are scattered in the literature, they need pulling together under some framework such as that provided by the rational choice or decision perspective (see Clarke and Cornish, 1985; Cornish and Clarke, 1986). From this prespective, suicide is seen as an intentional act (Halbwachs, 1978; Baechler, 1975), the outcome of a decision made with varying degrees of rationality and determination to end a life without hope (Beck et al., 1975; Farber, 1968).

In analyzing these decisions, account would need to be taken of accompanying psychiatric factors, such as alcoholism, which is frequently encountered among suicides, and of depression, which seems to lead to crude "either/or" thinking and to pessimistic evaluations of alternative courses of action (Brandt, 1975; Shneidman, 1985). Extreme ambivalence and superstitious thinking associated with a "gamble with death" have also often been described (Lester and Lester, 1971).[1] Finally, it would need to be recognized that a suicide decision is sometimes fully rational (Battin and Mayo, 1980).

Though the main focus of theoretical analysis is the thought processes underlying the suicidal decision, the motivational and situational contexts are also important. The source of the motive for suicide may not be especially problematic, since this might be any of the misfortunes and miseries of the human condition; rather, the method of dealing with motivating factors seems to be at issue. Contributing to thoughts and feelings, and ultimately to the choice of a solution, will be aspects of the situation unrelated to the source of unhappiness or distress. Chief among these may be features of the individual's daily life that could impede or facilitate suicide, such as the availability of an acceptable mean of death.

This represents the merest sketch of a theory, but some of the main implications should already be apparent:

1. From this perspective, suicide is seen as the outcome of a dynamic interplay between objective motivating and facilitating conditions and the individual's thoughts and feelings.
2. Suicidal thoughts are sometimes quite transitory and may not be experienced again by a particular individual. Moreover, lethality of intent might vary along a continuum for the same individual at different times.
3. Nothing is assumed about the pathology of the behavior. In many cases the decision to commit suicide is readily understandable to other, whereas in other cases the underlying reasoning may appear to be greatly distorted to observers (even leaving aside clearly psychotic suicides).
4. Suicide is seen less as a unitary behavior than a collection of somewhat different behaviors distinguished by method, motivations, and populations involved.
5. No allegiance is owed to any single parent discipline. Both psychological and sociological motivating variables have their place, while the decision perspective has antecedents in economic analyses of suicide (Hamermesh and Soss, 1974).
6. Some previously puzzling features of suicide are more readily explicable from this view: for example that religious beliefs may protect their adherents from suicide, that newspaper accounts of suicides stimulate imitative waves of suicide (Phillips, 1974), and that certain locations serve as a magnet to the suicidally inclined.
7. Any attempt to explain the suicide rate of a country or a region needs to give as much attention to availability of lethal agents and the cultural

---

[1] These facts suggest a clear role for cognitive therapy in attempting to modify the thinking patterns of suicidal individuals (see Velkof and·Huberty, 1988).

acceptability of suicide as to such demographic and social factors as unemployment or alcoholism.

8. Finally, and most important in light of the present concerns, a decision perspective provides an understanding of the important causal role the choice-structuring properties of different methods play in suicide and, in particular, of why wholesale displacement to other lethal methods of suicide does not typically occur after a particular method for suicide is restricted.

A Public Health Approach to Prevention

In Chapter 1 we identified the two primary approaches to preventing suicide as being the establishment of suicide prevention centers and the psychiatric treatment of depression through drugs and therapy. At best, the success of these methods has been limited, and other promising approaches should be tried, including controlling the availability of lethal agents. Measures of this kind discussed earlier include stiffer gun control laws, elimination of carbon monoxide from public gas supplies and car exhausts, barriers or reduced public access at notorious jumps sites, restrictions on the sale of poisonous substances, and measures designed to prevent overdoses with medicines.

As a secondary and supportive strategy to instituting controls on lethal agents, we advocate attempting to manipulate the acceptability of suicide as a solution to life's problems (for example, by emphasizing the possible costs of a failure in terms of permanent disability or disfigurement) and reducing the kinds of publicity more likely to influence the suggestible. The empirical base for these suggestions is less firm; they derive partly from our belief, buttressed by the decision perspective on suicide, that the opportunity structure for suicide is more than just a matter of the physical availability of lethal agents. Possibly of equal importance is the individual's perception of suicide as a solution to his problems. This perception is influenced by a composite of attitudes and beliefs about suicide as an act, including the person's feelings about different ways of committing suicide. It is to these subjective components of the opportunity structure that our supplementary proposal is primarily addressed.

Before discussing these proposals in more depth, we should note that they fall under the rubric of a public health approach. Winslow (1923) characterized this many years ago as preventing disease, prolonging life, and promoting health by doing the following: sanitizing the environment, controlling communicable diseases, educating people in personal hygiene, organizing medical services for diagnosing and preventing disease, and improving the standard of living so that good health can be maintained.

The broad scope of this definition helps to explain why our proposals differ significantly from some other "public health" measures for preventing suicide suggested by Oast and Zitrin (1974) and by Welu (1972). Oast and

Zitrin's proposals were concerned with the provision of better service and care for attempters and Welu's primarily with more active progams to identify and reach out to individuals in the community at risk for suicide. Our own approach is closer to those of Browning (1974a), who was concerned mainly with establishing procedures to prevent the sale of handguns to individuals at risk for suicide; Brown (1979), who, while acknowledging the need for more deliberate efforts to diagnose and treat depression, primarily advocated reducing lethal means; and Seiden (1977), who in a brief article deals comprehensively with issues relating to reducing the availability and lethality of the agents of suicide.

Suicide-Proofing the Environment

We have sought to provide increased empirical and theoretical support for the idea—current for some time in the journals—that reducing the opportunities for suicide will lower the suicide rate. It has not been our intention to develop detailed preventive proposal, since this would require not only more research, but also expertise that we do not possess. To make realistic proposals for restrictions on the prescribing of dangerous drugs, for example, or on their supply and packaging would require specialized knowledge of medicine and the pharamaceutical industry. Cost-benefit studies (requiring economic expertise) may also have to be undertaken, as well as surveys of prescribing policies and patients' ingesting practices. The same holds for developing detailed proposals to restrict any other lethal agent. Nevertheless, we attempt here to draw lessons from existing research for the control of poisons and drugs, guns, carbon monoxide, and jump sites. With the exception of the latter, these are common agents of suicide that, between them, account for the majority of suicidal deaths in many countries.

We should first, however, identify some of the constraints and opportunities that define the scope of this approach to prevention.

Constraints and Opportunities

The first, and perhaps most important, constraint is that, despite the official government position, suicide prevention has limited public appeal. Unless it involves youngsters, the responsibility for suicide is usually seen to rest with the individual or his family rather than with society. There is also little appreciation of the economic costs to the community, in terms of ambulance and hospital care, of investigations by police and coroner, the loss of a productive taxpayer, and the need for a family to be placed on welfare. The public is therefore unlikely to accept that the economic costs of emission controls or detoxification of the gas supply, for example, are justified by a reduction in deaths by suicide. And social costs in terms of inconvenience to the public or the erosion of civil liberties continues to militate against gun controls and reduced access to some jump sites. (For a well-documented example, see McWilliam's [1936] account of the campaign to install barriers on the Arroyo Seco Bridge in Pasadena.)

Even where the need for reducing access to lethal agents is accepted in principle, it may still be argued that the difficulty of reducing opportunities for traditional forms of suicide (cutting, drowning, and hanging) limits the applicability of this approach. It may further be held that, with the exception of gun controls, most of the likely gains have already been made—domestic gas in the Unied States is largely nontoxic already and soon all vehicles will be unusable for suicide.

A final source of resistance is the continuing concern about displacement. Even when it is accepted that displacement may not be immediate, it may be held that "delayed displacement" or "innovation" (Chapter 6) will eventually result in the substitution and use of some new method of suicide.

To deal with these points in reverse order, even if some delayed displacement does occur, many lives may be saved in the meantime, and the eventual displacement may be to less lethal methods. This would lead to an additional saving of lives, as only a few of those who survive a suicide attempt go on subsequently to kill themselves. (Seiden, 1977, reported that only 4 percent of more than 700 individuals prevented from jumping off the Golden Gate Bridge subsequently committed suicide within a follow-up period of more than 20 years.)

As for the supposedly limited application of the approach, even if it is difficult to reduce opportunities for traditional forms of suicide, these include some of the less successful methods, such as cutting and drowning (Card, 1974). As such they demand less urgent attention. In addition, the possible role of the safety razor in the decline of cutting suicides should not be overlooked, and Burvill (1980) may be correct in suggesting that drowning as a method of suicide has declined in Australia and other Western countries as a result of more people being able to swim. ["It would take a very marked and sustained determination for a person who can swim well to suicide by drowning" (p. 266).] Moreover, to suggest that little more may be gained by further blocking opportunities is excessively optimistic (surely further important gains can be made at least with overdoses and jump sites) and ignores two important facts. First, technology is constantly changing, which may bring both new opportunities to commit suicide and new means of prevention. Second, some other countries have yet to solve their gas suicide and poisoning problems. For example, countries such as India, Sri Lanka, and Malaysia would benefit from restrictions on pesticides, which are the major agents of suicide in these countries (see Chapter 6).

One way of dealing with the apparent public indifference to suicide may be to link its prevention with some other benefits. For example, gun controls are also likely to reduce homicidal and accidental deaths, and emission controls benefit the environment. Issues of inconvenience to the public or erosion of civil liberties may need to be resolved through some kind of Benthamite calculus. For example, if Seiden and Spence (1983–84) are correct in arguing that the much greater risk of suicide from the Golden Gate Bridge compared with the Bay Bridge is due partly to the latter's restricted pedestrian access, and if costs or aesthetic considerations really do prohibit the fitting of effective antisuicide barriers on the Golden Gate Bridge, then might not the sacrifice involved in foregoing walks across the bridge by a relatively few people be justified by the saving of some lives? Pursuit of this line might sometimes require the assistance of the law. Thus, relatives of suicides might bring suits against authorities, such as those responsible for particular bridges, who fail to take necessary precautions.

Finally, it may also be possible to identify cheaper alternative means of reducing availability as suggested, for example, in our following discussion of carbon monoxide. That many routes to successful prevention exist has been demonstrated by Haddon (1973) in the field of injury prevention.[2] He has developed a schema consisting of 10 strategies for modifying a hazard, which include preventing its creation in the first place (e.g., prohibiting manufacture of handguns) and separating it in time or space from those to be protected (e.g., statutory limits on gun ownership). Examples of potential applications of Haddon's strategies, reproduced with some modifications in Table 8.1, have been developed for suicide by Gerberich et al. (1985).

Carbon monoxide

Perhaps the domestic gas supply is still toxic only where it would be too expensive to supply natural gas. It might still be possible to save lives, however, by redesigning appliances. We suggested in Chapter 2 that the comparatively low rate of domestic gas suicide in the Netherlands before detoxification may have been due to the design of the gas cookers and fires. Ovens had downward-opening doors and the flame of gas fires was enclosed behind a glass door. In the United States, devices to turn off the gas automatically if the flame extinguished were installed. In general, any design measures that make it more difficult for potential suicides to gain access to the toxic gas would be worth considering.

On the other hand, few countries have as strict controls on car exhaust

---

[2] From a public health perspective the link between suicides and accidents may be closer than is usually thought. Both are causes of death rather than diseases, as traditionally conceived in the public health model. Indeed, they appear together in the International Classification of Diseases. A general conclusion from the accident prevention literature (Barry, 1975) is that efforts to persuade people to take precautions are less productive than legal compulsions (see the literature on seat belt use) and that neither strategy is as successful as environmental change (e.g., passive restraints, such as airbags).

Table 8.1. Haddon's injury prevention stategies applied to suicide.

Haddon's strategies	Examples of potential applications in the prevention of suicide
1. To prevent the creation of the hazard in the first place *or*	Limit the manufacture and/or distribution of firearms; Develop safer means of self-protection
2. To reduce the amount of the hazard brought into being	
3. To prevent the release of the hazard that already exists	Ban gun sales in certain populations
4. To modify the rate or spatial distribution of release of the hazard that already exists	Package tablets individually to prevent rapid consumption; supply them only in suppository form; use judicious prescribing
5. To separate in time, or in space, the hazard and what is being protected	Separate the ammunition from guns; separate drugs by use of a locked cupboard
6. To separate the hazard from that which is to protected by interposition of a material barrier	Utilize fences/barriers on bridges and high buildings to prevent impulsive suicidal acts
7. To modify relevant basic qualities of the hazard	Alter pharmacologic agents to reduce side effects of drug ingestion
8. To make what is to be protected more resistant to damage from hazard	Institute training in swimming; Make suicide seem less acceptable
9. To begin to counter damage already done *and*	Improve emergency services
10. To stabilize and repair the object.	

Source: Adapted from Gerberich et al., 1985.

emissions as exist in the United States, though some European countries, persuaded by environmental concerns, are now enacting controls. In time, therefore, the problem of car exhaust suicides might be greatly reduced, if not eliminated. Where economic or other reasons stand in the way of emission controls, some lives might be saved through minor modifications to the exhaust pipes of cars to increase the difficulty of connecting a hose. (A recent Swedish study [Thorson et al., 1988] showed that 74 percent of car exhaust suicides used a hose connected to the exhaust pipe.) Alternatively, it might be possible to install devices to switch off the engine when it has been left idling for more than a few minutes or when carbon monoxide levels rise to a dangerous level in the passenger compartment—measures that would also have environmental benefits.

Jump Sites

Seiden and Spence (1983–84) have noted that suicide deaths have been greatly reduced by the installation of safety barriers at some notorious sites formerly accounting for hundreds of deaths, such as the Eiffel Tower, Mt. Mihara, and the Arroyo Seco Bridge in Pasadena. The survivors of jumps from the Golden Gate Bridge interviewed by Rosen (1975) were unanimous in supporting the installation of antisuicide barriers, saying that these would have prevented their attempts. Objections to such measures usually center on the costs and unsightlines of such barriers, but it seems likely that ways around these difficulties could be found.

Costs may not allow all high buildings to be suicide-proofed. Those that are air-conditioned, however, may require only restricted access to the roof and barriers around stairwells. For others, stops to prevent windows from being opened wide may prevent accidents as well as suicide. In general, buildings with free access to the public may require a higher standard of safety, although any building that begins to attract jumpers should be given attention before it becomes notorious.

Each year, small but significant numbers of people kill themselves by jumping under trains, particularly in the subway (Guggenheim and Weisman, 1972), while a number of other fall accidentally. On the London Underground, for example, about five people per month end up beneath trains (Taylor, 1982), some of whom survive but with terrible injuries. Especially for the subway systems being planned, costs may not prohibit designing platforms for which trains are accessible only through doors like those on elevators, or as at Gatwick Airport in the United Kingdom.

Poisons and Drugs

We have already mentioned the potential in a number of countries for control of agricultural pesticides. More economically developed countries may have considerable potential for tighter controls on dangerous drugs. There are three main approaches: controls on prescribing (such as have been introduced in many countries for barbiturates); changes in the means of packaging, storing, and administering drugs (see Siegel and Siegel, 1981); and the development of safer alternative drugs.

In Chapter 6, we documented some notable success of prescribing controls,and this approach will undoubtedly have a continuing role when linked with analysis of the changes in the drugs used for suicide. However, not all dangerous drugs can be obtained only by prescription. For example, paracetomol (found in Tylenol in the United States) is now a favored agent of suicide in Scotland. McMurray et al. (1987) have made the intriguing suggestion that its greater use reflects the widespread perception that it has fewer unwelcome side effects than some alternatives such as aspirin! This leads them to propose that "education of the general public to the dangers of paracetomol (or any drug) might greatly discourage its use in self-poisoning."

For nonprescription drugs, individual packaging of tablets may play a role in preventing highly impulsive suicides (Edwards and Whitlock, 1968; Fox, 1975),[3] though Gazzard et al. (1976) and Poore (1976), an industry spokesman, are skeptical of this approach. To us it seems intuitively no less valuable a measure than one adopted by the Japanese authorities in dealing with the epidemic of suicides at Mt. Mihara (Chapter 7): they forbad the sale of one-way tickets on the ferry to the island where the volcano is located (Ellis and Allen, 1961). Presumably the purchase of a one-way ticket might reinforce the resolution of waiverers to take their own lives.

Far greater potential appears to exist, however, for the development and preferential use of safer alternative drugs, such as the antidepressant Tolvon (Hepburn, 1980). In this regard, analyses such as those undertaken by Henry (1988) of the "fatal toxicity indices" of different antidepressants (see Table 6.1) have a very important role to play not only in guiding prescription practices, but also in encouraging the pharmaceutical companies to devote greater effort to the search for safe drugs.

Guns

Guns demand urgent attention for two reasons: their increasing use for suicide in the United States (see Table 4.1) and their comparative deadlines. Thus, in Card's (1974) sample, 92 percent of suicide attempts by firearm were successful, compared with 78 percent for carbon monoxide, 9 percent for other gases, 78 percent for hanging, 67 percent for drowning, 23 percent for poisoning, and 4 percent for cutting. Even if reduced gun availability resulted in displacement to other methods of suicide, lives would be saved because these alternatives are generally less lethal.

Given the widespread public support for gun ownership, further gun controls will not be accepted simply in the interests of preventing suicide. Resistance to gun control has been strong even when the goal was a reduction in violent crime. However, when accidents, suicides, and homicides are

---

[3] "Twenty to thirty tablets or capsules of barbiturate sedatives supplied in a bottle can be tipped out and swallowed with water very quickly. It takes about a minute to extract six to eight aspirin tablets in a calm, methodical manner from their cellophane or tinfoil wrappings....We would guess that the time required to prepare a lethal dose in this fashion would be quite sufficient to permit tempers to cool and wiser counsels to prevail." (Edwards and Whitlock, 1968, p. 993.)

taken together, the resulting annual toll of deaths is very large. Treating this as a major public health problem may garner more support for controls, though much still depends on trends in crime and the perceived need for self-defense.

Proponents of gun control might receive support from two unexpected quarters. The first of these is from women, traditionally opposed to violence, whose political and economic power is increasing year by year. (Indeed, Zimring and Hawkins [1978] have suggestd that "Perhaps in searching for the eventual solution to the American handgun stalemate, we should redirect our attention from the *New York Times* to the *Ladies Home Journal*," p. 188.) The second is from taxpayers when they learn about the tremendous costs of treating gunshot wounds. Based on a study of a sample of patients with gunshot wounds admitted to San Francisco General Hospital, Martin et al. (1988) have recently estimated that the nationwide costs of treating firearm injuries may be more than $1 billion per year. Of the average cost of $6915 per patient in their sample, 85.6 percent was borne by taxpayer, while private sources paid only 14.4 percent. As the authors comment: "[When] considering bills to restrict the availability of handguns ... legislators must be aware that the issue is not simply one of individual rights, since taxpayers pay most of the costs associated with firearm injuries." These findings support the idea of instituting a tax on guns so that gun owners rather than the general taxpayer pay, not only for victim compensation as suggested by (Bonney, 1985), but also for the considerable costs of treating those wounded by guns.

Although much can be gained by treating gun availability as a public health issue, it should not be forgotten that effective measures for suicide may not be effective for accidents and crime. For example, long guns may play a greater role in accidents while handguns play a larger part in suicide and crime (Lester and Carke, in preparation). This means that, whatever their value in relation to suicide and crime, increased handgun controls may do little to reduce accidents. Again, restrictions on the *carrying* of handguns are more likely to reduce crime than suicide (see Chapter 5).

Another approach that should be pursued more vigorously is to take the manufacturers of guns and ammunition to court. Although the courts have thrown out liability suits from the relatives of murder victims against gun manufacturers on the basis that the design, manufacture, and marketing of handguns constitutes a dangerous activity (Bonney, 1985; Smith, 1987), the possibility of suing manufacturers of Saturday night specials has been raised by the ruling in *Kelly* v. *R.G. Industries* (Lippman, 1986). Gun manufacturers can also be sued for defective products, including inadequate safety devices and warnings (Dillon, 1984; Goff, 1984).

It is also possible to sue murderers who use guns and those who aid and abet them (Forrester, 1984). Recently, a pawnshop that sold a gun used for murder settled out of court for $1.9 million and stopped selling handguns (Anon, 1987). However, in a recent case, courts held that the use of a stolen gun for murder did not render the owner liable (*Romero* v. *NRA*, DDC 1980, 749 F2d). (Ironically in this case, the gun was stolen from the headquarters of the National Rifle Association and was illegally owned by an employee there.)

The importance of legal suits against the manufacturers, sellers, and owners of guns is that no matter how many claims are thrown out of court, it is always possible that one suit, based perhaps on different premises, may be upheld. As soon as the first suit is won and upheld, the floodgates could open.

Reducing Acceptability and Suggestion

There is an interesting contrast between public health education concerning medical diseases and that concerning suicide. In educating the public about smoking, for example, public health information has focused on its dangers. The facts that smoking causes lung cancer and may damage the embryos of pregnant women are stressed. A recent television advertisement featured Yul Bryner, the film star, who made a videotape before his death from lung cancer urging people "Don't Smoke!" Those opposed to smoking have published shocking photographs of diseased lung tissue and heart-rending stories about those who have suffered from lung cancer. Similarly, AIDS education focuses on the dangers of contracting AIDS through certain forms of sexual behavior. Strategies to reduce the risk of contracting AIDS are mentioned, including use of condoms and avoidance of casual and anal sex.

Leaving aside their smaller scale, public education programs on suicide have been very different in character. They have generally focused on identifying clues in people who are considering suicide and acquainting people with local suicide prevention and crisis intervention agencies. The value of such information is unknown and it is at least possible, as argued by Lester (1972b), that advertising about suicide prevention centers may actually increase a community's suicide rate. Documented claims of an increase in adolescent suicides have occasionally followed the presentation on television of real-life dramas involving suicidal teenagers (Gould and Shaffer, 1986).

Aside from this possibility, it is clear that this approach is very different from those for smoking and AIDS because information is omitted that would arouse anxiety and make people think twice before attempting suicide. When a person dying from AIDS is presented on television, it does not seem to encourage viewers to find a way of contracting the disease. When a report of suicide is presented, however, people apparently are often persuaded to kill themselves, especially if the subject is as famous as Marilyn Monroe or Ernest Hemingway (Stack, 1987).

Can public information about suicide be changed to increase the chances of deterring suicide? Here are some suggestions:

1. Many people survive suicide attempts with terrible and permanent disabilities, a fact which is not generally known. For example, the effects of carbon monoxide poisoning include apathy, confusion, and memory defects. In many patients these symptoms clear up in two years, but some patients suffer permanent mental impairment (Kolb and Brodie, 1982). Similarly, some people survive gunshot wounds, jumping in front of trains and subway cars, and jumps from bridges and buildings. Many of these survivors suffer severe injuries and remain permanently handicapped (Westermeyer, 1984). Even the relatively painless methods of ingesting medications can have severe consequences. An overdose of paracetamol, for example, may lead to severe kidney damage, leaving the survivors of suicide attempts in need of continual medical treatment. And a fact that may deter teenage girls, for example, is that drugs taken in overdose can sometimes lead to a loss of bowel control.

2. A growing body of work is appearing on the difficulties faced by survivors of suicide. Their anger and guilt are much more difficult to cope with than that felt after a natural death, and the survivors often face hostility from neighbors and friends (Rudestam and Imbroll, 1983). Indeed, it is common to find the children of suicides later committing suicide too. Leicester Hemingway killed himself, many years after his father and his brother Ernest had done so (Lester, 1988a). The American poet John Berryman was only 12 when his father committed suicide, and he too later killed himself. Public education could focus on the grief and suffering caused to relatives and friends by those who commit suicide.

3. Many religions stigmatize suicide, some more strongly than others. The Christian religion in particular views suicide as a sin. Muslims also have very low rates of suicide since the action is frowned on in most circumstances. One way to reduce the acceptability of suicide may be to focus attention on this moral disapproval of suicide.

4. Clearly there are dangers of interfering with the freedom of the press, but David Phillips (Phillips and Carstensen, 1988), a pioneer in the study of suggestion and suicide (see Chapter 7), has recently suggested some ways of altering the treatment of suicide in the media. The purpose would be to reduce the publicity accorded to suicide stories and to change the manner in which the suicide story is reported. These suggestions include more discussion of the costs of suicide, mentioned earlier, but also considering the suicide story as a type of "natural advertisement," the effect of which would be reduced if treated in the following way:

If the advertisement is not repeated. Thus, suicide stories (or advertisements) appearing on a single program seem to have a smaller effect than multiprogram stories or advertisements.... If the advertisement is placed in an obscure location. Cover-page advertisements in magazines are more expensive because they are thought to be more effective. Similarly, Phillips (unpublished research) found that front-page suicide stories had a detectable effect, whereas inside-page stories did not.... If the characters in the advertisement are presented in a neutral or unsympathetic light. People are probably less likely to imitate a character in an advertisement (or suicide story) if it is difficult to identify with him or her.... If the advertisement mentions alternatives to the advertised product. Commercial advertisements never mention competing products (unless with the intent of disparaging them). It is interesting to note that the "natural advertisement" of a suicide story often has the same monolithic character: The story focuses on one response to psychological anguish—suicide—without indicating that there are many other possible responses as well. It is possible that mention of these alternatives (hotlines, counseling, self-help groups, etc.) in the suicide story would reduce the tendency to imitative suicide. (p. 111)

Conclusions

As mentioned in the Preface, our goal has been to convince public health officials and others that restricting lethal agents—closing exits to suicide— should take its place, alongside crisis intervention and the psychiatric treatment of depression, as a third major strategy for suicide prevention. Steps to the achieving this goal include provision of (1) clear evidence that availability of lethal agents is directly related to the extent of their use in suicide, (2) evidence that gains achieved by reducing availability are not simply lost through displacement, (3) an explanation of the conditions under which displacement occurs, (4) a model of suicide that adequately encompasses the role of situational opportunities in causation, (5) enough practical suggestions for controlling lethal agents to serve as the basis for a well-rounded policy initiative, and (6) a start in identifying the constraints and opportunities that will determine the practical scope of such a policy.

As to the first of these requirements, we believe the evidence is now incontestable that the availability of a lethal agent is related to its use in suicide. This has been shown for guns, drugs, carbon monoxide, jump sites, and a variety of other means of death. This is not to say that the evidence is all of equal quality or that more research is not needed. On the contrary, preventive action is unlikely to be taken with respect to drugs and firearms without fuller evidence of the role played in suicide by their easy availability. Concerning drugs, detailed studies of the rate of overdose deaths associated with different products would be of inestimable value, while for guns more detailed information about patterns of ownership, particularly for the individual states of the United States, is urgently needed.

The evidence on displacement is more mixed. Most studies (the strongest being that of the detoxification of the gas supply in England and Wales) suggest that although some displacement is inevitable, it is far from complete. It is unlikely that much more will be learned simply by repeating statistical studies of patterns of suicide. We have suggested that more research is needed into the choice-structuring properties of different methods of suicide by questioning samples of people, especially the suicide-prone, about their attitudes toward the use of these methods. Research of this sort should assist understanding of the reasons why displacement may not be inevitable and may also help in predicting when it is more or less likely to occur. Further development of the "decision" theory of suicide, which we discussed only in outline but which emphasizes the importance of the individual's thinking processes and the situational context in which decisions are made, might also assist.

In addition, the decision theory might guide the direction of the research needed to establish a firmer basis for the supplementary preventive strategy we have proposed, that of reducing suggestion and the acceptability of suicide. The empirical evidence supporting this strategy is much weaker, despite the impressive studies undertaken by Phillips and others. Although we believe there are already sufficient grounds for experimenting with this strategy, more will have to be learned about the mechanisms by which religious prohibitions are internalized and the circumstances under which people are most suggestible before its likely scope can be assessed.

There is no doubt, however, that there is a full agenda of policy work to be undertaken to reduce the availability of a variety of lethal agents. The discouraging history of gun control in the criminal justice arena shows how much there is to be done about this lethal agent alone, though greater progress may follow from treating the widespread availability of firearms as a broader problem of public health. Much also needs to be done in the United States to institute more effective controls on a variety of medications. In other countries, controls are needed not only on guns and medicines, but also on pesticides, exhaust gases, and toxic domestic gas. Efforts to impose these controls will lead to a demand for new kinds of research to identify the most cost-effective and acceptable solutions. In other words, for public health professionals and researchers alike, there is a full program for the foreseeable future to close more of the exits to suicide.

References

Achte, K.A., and Lonnqvist, J. Suicide in Finnish culture. *Suicide in different cultures*, edited by Norman L. Farberow. Baltimore: University Park Press, 1975.

Adelstein, A., and Mardon, C. Suicides 1961–1974. *Population Trends*, 1975, 2(Winter), 13–18.

Alvarez, A. *The savage god.* New York: Random House, 1971.

Anon. Shop that sold gun to pay $1.9 million. *Philadelphia Inquirer*, 1987, May 8, 16a.

Auerbach, S., and Kilmann, P. Crisis intervention. *Psychological Bulletin*, 1977, 84, 1189–1217.

Baechler, J. *Suicides.* New York: Basic Books, 1975.

Bagley, C. The evaluation of a suicide prevention scheme by an ecological method. *Social Science and Medicine*, 1968, 2, 1–14.

Bakal, C. *No right to bear arms.* New York: Paperback Library, 1968.

Barraclough, B.M. Suicide prevention, recurrent affective disorder and lithium. *British Journal of Psychiatry*, 1972, 121, 391–392.

Barraclough, B.M., Jennings, C., and Moss, J.R. Suicide prevention by the Samaritans. *Lancet*, 1977, i, 237–239.

Barraclough, B.M., Nelson, B., Bunch, J., and Sainsbury, P. Suicide and barbiturate prescribing. *Journal of the Royal College of General Practitioners*, 1971, 21, 645–653.

Barry, P.Z. Individual versus community orientation in the prevention of injuries. *Preventive Medicine*, 1975, 4, 47–56.

Battin, M.P., and Mayo, D.J. *Suicide: The philosophical issues.* London: Peter Owen, 1980.

Beck, A.T., Kovacs, M., and Weissman, A. Hopelessness and suicidal behavior. *Journal of the American Medical Association*, 1975, 234, 1146–1149.

Berger, L.R. Suicides and pesticides in Sri Lanka. *American Journal of Public Health*, 1988, 78, 826–828.

Blum, R. Contemporary threats to adolescent health in the United States. *Journal of the American Medical Association*, 1987, 257, 3390–3395.

Bonney, P.R. Manufacturers' strict liability for handgun injury. *Georgetown Law Journal*, 1985, 73, 1437–1463.

Boor, M. Methods of suicide and implications for suicide prevention. *Journal of Clinical Psychology*, 1981, 37, 75, 70.

Boyd, J.H. The increasing rate of suicide by firearms. *New England Journal of Medicine*, 1983, 308, 872–874.

Brandt, R.B. The rationality of suicide. In S. Perlin (ed.) *A handbook for the study of suicide*. London: Oxford University Press, 1975.

Brewer, C., and Farmer, R.D.T. Self-poisoning in 1984: A prediction that didn't come true. *British Medical Journal*, 1985, 290, 391.

Bridge, T., Potkin, S., Zung, W., and Soldo, B. Suicide prevention centers. *Journal of Nervous and Mental Disease*, 1977, 164, 18–24.

Brown, J.M. Suicides in Britain. *Archives of General Psychiatry*, 1979, 36, 1119–1124.

Browning, C.H. Suicide, firearms and public health. *American Journal of Public Health*, 1974a, 64, 313–316.

Browning, C.H. Epidemiology of suicide: Firearms. *Comprehensive Psychiatry*, 1974b, 15, 549–553.

Bulusu, L., and Alderson, M. Suicides, 1950–1982. *Population Trends*, 1984, 35, 11–17.

Burvill, P.W. Changing patterns of suicide in Australia, 1910–1977. *Acta Psychiatrica Scandinavia*, 1980, 62, 258–268.

Butscher, E. *Sylvia Plath*. New York: Seabury, 1976.

Card, J.J. Lethality of suicidal methods and suicide risk: Two distinct concepts. *Omega*, 1974, 5, 37–45.

Centers for Disease Control. *Youth suicide in the United States, 1970–1980*. Atlanta: Centers for Disease Controlj, 1986.

Clarke, M.J. Suicides by opium and its derivatives in England and Wales. *Psychological Medicine*, 1985, 15, 237–242.

Clarke, R.V. Displacement: An old problem in new perspective. In G. Saville, and D. Morley (eds.), *Research futures in environmental criminology*. Toronto: ABL, in press.

Clarke, R.V., and Cornish, D.B. Modelling offenders' decisions. In M. Tonry and N. Morris (eds.). *Crime and Justice*, Vol. 6, Chicago: University of Chicago Press, 1985, pp. 147–185.

Clarke, R.V. and Jones, P. Suicide and increased availability of handguns in the United States. *Social Science and Medicine*, 1989, 28, 805–809.

Clarke, R.V., and Lester, D. Toxicity of car exhausts and opportunity for suicide: Comparison between Britain and the United States. *Journal of Epidemiology and Community Health*, 1987, 41, 114–120.

Clarke, R.V. and Mayhew, P.M. *Designing out crime*, London: Her Majesty's Stationary Office, 1980.

Clarke, R.V., and Mayhew, P. The British gas suicide story and its criminological implications. In M. Tonry and N. Morris (eds.). *Crime and Justice*, Vol. 10, 1988, Chicago: University of Chicago Press, pp. 79–116.

Clarke, R.V., and Mayhew, P. Crime as opportunity: A note on domestic gas suicide in Britain and the Netherlands. *British Journal of Criminology*, 1989, 29, 35–46.

Cook, P.J. The role of firearms in violent crime. In M.E. Wolfgang and N.A. Weiner (eds.). *Criminal violence*. Beverly Hills: Sage, 1982, pp. 236–291.

Cornish, D.B., and Clarke, R.V. *The reasoning criminal*. New York: Springer-Verlag, 1986.

Cornish D.B., and Clarke, R.V. Crime specialisation, crime displacement and rational choice theory. In H. Wegener, F. Losel and J. Haish (eds), *Criminal behavior and the justice system: Psychological perspectives*. New York: Springer-Verlag, 1989.

Danto, B.L. Firearm suicide in the home setting. *Omega*, 1972, 3, 111–119.

Danto, B.L. A discussion about gun control as a practical means of homicide and suicide prevention. *Proceedings of the 10th International Congress for Suicide Prevention*. Ottawa: IASP, 1979, 1–8.

Dillon, M. Hitting the mark. *Santa Clara Law Review*, 1984, 24, 743–762.

Drinker, C.W. *Carbon monoxide asphyxia*. New York: Oxford University Press, 1938.

Dublin, L. *Suicide: A sociological and statistical study*. New York: Ronald Press, 1963.

Dublin, L., and Bunzel, B. *To be or not to be*. New York: Harrison Smith, 1933.

Durkheim, E. *Le suicide*. Paris: Alcan, 1897.

Edwards, J.E. and Whitlock, F.A. Suicide and attempted suicide in Brisbane. *Medical Journal of Australia*, 1968, 2, 989–995.

Elliott, C. *The history of the natural gas conversion in Great Britain*. Royston, Cambridge: Cambridge Information and Research Service, 1980.

Ellis, E.R., and Allen, G.N. *Traitor within: Our suicide problem*. Garden City, NY: Doubleday, 1961.

Farber, M.L. *Theory of suicide*. New York: Funk & Wagnalls, 1968.

Farberow, N.L. and Shneidman, E.S. *The cry for help*. New York: McGraw-Hill, 1961.

Farberow, N.L., and Simon, M.D. Suicides in Los Angeles and Vienna. *Public Health Reports*, 1969, 84, 389–403.

Farmer, R.D.T. Suicide by different methods. *Postgraduate Medical Journal*, 1979, 775–779.

Farmer, R.D.T. The relationship between suicide and parasuicide. In R. Farmer and S. Hirsch (eds.). *The suicide syndrome*. London: Croom Helm, 1980.

Farmer, R.D.T., and Rohde, J.R. Effect of availability and acceptability of lethal instruments on suicide mortality. *Acta Psychiatrica Scandinavia*, 1980, 62, 436–446.

Federal Highway Administration. *Highway Statistics, 1980*. Washington, DC: U.S. Government Printing Office, 1982.

Forrester, D.J. Halberstam v Welch. *American Journal of Trial Advocacy*, 1984, 7, 377–384.

Fox, R. The suicide drop—why? *Royal Society of Health Journal*, 1975, 95, 9–20.

Friedman, G. Suicide and the altered prescription. *New York State Medical Journal*, 1966, 66, 3005–3007.

Friedman, P. Suicide among police: A study of 93 suicides among New York City Policemen, 1934–1940. In E. S. Shneidman (ed.). *Essays on self-destruction*. New York: Science House, 1967.

Gabor, T. Crime displacement: The literature and strategies for its investigation. *Crime and Justice*, 1978, 6, 100–106.

Gazzard, B.G., David, M., Spooner, J.B., and Williams, R.S. Why paracetamol? *Journal of International Medical Research*, 1976, 4 (Suppl 4), 25–31.

Geisel, M., Roll, R., and Wettick, R. The effectiveness of state and local regulation of handguns. *Duke Law Journal*, 1969, 647–673.

Gerberich, S.G., Hays, M., Mandel J.S., Gibson R.W., and Van der Heide, C.J.

Analysis of suicides in adolescents and young adults: Implications for prevention. In U. Laaser, R. Senault, and H. Viefhues (eds.). *Primary health care in the making*. Berlin, Heidelberg: Springer-Verlag, 1985.

Gibbs, W.T., and Arnold, A.R.G. Rise and fall of suicide rates in Australia. *Medical Journal of Australia*, 1972, 2, 1149–1150.

Goff, A.K. Defective firearms. *Trial*, 1984, 20(11), 36–40.

Gould, M.S., and Shaffer, D. The impact of suicide in television movies. *New England Journal of Medicine*, 1986, 315, 690–694.

Guggenheim, F.G., and Weisman, A.D. Suicide in the subway. *Journal of Nervous and Mental Disease*, 1972, 155, 404–409.

Haddon, W. Jr. Energy damage and the ten countermeasure strategies. *Journal of Trauma*, 1973, 13, 321–331.

Halbwachs, M. *The causes of suicides*. London: Routledge & Kegan Paul, 1978.

Hamermesh, D., and Soss, N. An economic theory of suicide. *Journal of Political Economics*, 1974, 82, 83–98.

Harding, R. *Firearms and violence in Australian life*. Nedlands: University of Western Australia Press, 1981.

Hassall, C., and Trethowan, W.M. Suicide in Birmingham. *British Medical Journal*, 1972 (March 18), 717–718.

Hay, P., and Bornstein, R. Failed suicide by emission gas poisoning. *American Journal of Psychiatry*, 1984, 141, 592–593.

Henderson, S., and Williams, C. On the prevention of suicide. *Australian and New Zealand Journal of Psychiatry*, 1974, 8, 237–240.

Henry, A.F., and Short, J.F. *Suicide and homicide*. New York: Free Press, 1954.

Henry, J.A. Toxicity in overdose. In B.E. Leonard and S.W. Parker (eds.). *Current approaches: Risks/benefits of antidepressants*. Southampton: Duphat Medical Relations, 1988.

Hepburn, S. Suicide in Australia. *Australian and New Zealand Journal of Psychiatry*, 1980, 14, 152.

Hirsh, J. Methods and fashions of suicide. *Mental Hygiene*, 1960, 337–339.

Hudgens, R.W. (editorial). Preventing suicide. *New England Journal of Medicine*, 1983, 308, 897–898.

Jacobs, J.A. Phenomenological study of suicide notes. *Social Problems*, 1967, 15, 60–72.

Jacobs, J. *The moral justification of suicide*. Springfield, IL: Charles C Thomas, 1982.

Jennings, C., Barraclough, B., and Moss, J. Have the Samaritans lowered the suicide rate? *Psychological Medicine*, 1978, 8, 413–422.

Jones, E., and Ray, M. Handgun control. Unpublished manuscript, 1980.

Jones, E.E. The rocky road from acts to dispositions. *American Psychologist*, 1979, 34, 107–117.

Kelly, G.A. *The psychology of personal constructs*. New York: W. W. Norton, 1955.

Kessel, N. Self-poisoning. In E.S. Shneidman (ed.). *Essays in self-destruction*. New York: Science House, 1967.

Kim, J. *Statistical package for the social sciences*. New York: McGraw-Hill, 1975.

Kolb, L., and Brodie H.K. *Modern Clinical Psychiatry*. Philadelphia: W.B. Sauaders, 1982.

Kreitman, N. The coal gas story. *British Journal of Preventive and Social Medicine*, 1976, 30, 86–93.

Kreitman, N., Philips, A.E., Greer, S., and Bagley, C.R. Parasuicide. *British Journal of Psychiatry*, 1969, 115, 746–747.

Kreitman, N., and Platt, S. Suicide, unemployment, and domestic gas detoxification in Britain. *Journal of Epidemiology and Community Health*, 1984, 38, 1–6.

Landers, D. Unsuccessful suicide by carbon monoxide. *Western Journal of Medicine*, 1981, 135, 360–363.

Lester, D. *Why people kill themselves*. Springfield, IL: Charles C Thomas, 1972 (a).

Lester, D. The myth of suicide prevention. *Comprehensive Psychiatry*, 1972 (b), 13, 555–560.

Lester, D. Prevention of suicide. *Journal of the American Medical Association*, 1973 (a), 225, 992.

Lester, D. Suicide prevention centers and prevention of suicide. *New England Journal of Medicine*, 1973 (b), 289, 380.

Lester, D. Effect of suicide prevention centers on suicide rates in the United States. *Health Services Reports*, 1974 (a), 89, 37–39.

Lester, D. Suicide prevention centers. *Journal of the American Medical Association*, 1974 (b), 229, 394.

Lester, D. Suicide prevention by the Samaritans, *Social Science and Medicine*, 1980, 14A, 85.

Lester, D. The morality of counseling the suicidal person. *Journal of Counseling and Psychotherapy*, 1981, 4(1), 79–84.

Lester, D. *Why people kill themselves*. Springfield, IL: Charles C Thomas, 1983.

Lester, D. *Gun control*. Springfield, IL: Charles C Thomas, 1984.

Lester, D. Suicide, homicide and the quality of life. *Suicide and Life-Threatening Behavior*, 1986, 16, 389–392.

Lester, D. Availability of guns and the likelihood of suicide. *Sociology and Social Research*, 1987 (a), 71, 287–288.

Lester, D. An availability-acceptability theory of suicide, *Activitas Nervosa Superior*, 1987 (b), 29, 164–166.

Lester, D. *Suicide as a learned behavior*. Springfield, IL: Charles C Thomas, 1987 (c).

Lester, D. Living in the shadow. In R.I. Yufit (ed.). *Proceedings of the 20th Annual Conference*. Denver: American Association of Suicidology, 1988 (a), pp. 422–433.

Lester, D. Restricting the availability of guns as a strategy for preventing suicide. *Biology and Society*, 1988 (b), 5, 127–129.

Lester, D. The perception of different methods of suicide. *Journal of General Psychology*, 1988 (c), 115, 215–217.

Lester, D. A critical-mass theory of national suicide rates. *Suicide and Threatening Behavior*, 1988 (d), 18, 279–284.

Lester, D. Youth suicide: A cross-cultural perspective. *Adolescence*, 1988 (e), 23, 955–958.

Lester, D. Why do people choose particular methods for suicide? *Activitas Nervosa Superior*, 1988 (f), 30, 312–314.

Lester, D. Gun ownership and suicide in the United States. *Psychological Medicine*, in press.

Lester, D., and Clarke, R.V. Effects of reduced toxicity of car exhaust. *American Journal of Public Health*, 1988, 78, 594.

Lester, D., and Clarke, R.V. The influence of firearm ownership on accidental deaths, in preparation.

Lester, D., and Frank, M.L. The use of motor vehicle exhaust for suicide and the availability of cars. *Acta Psychiatrica Scandinavia*, 1989, 79, 238–240.

Lester, G., and Lester, D. *Suicide: The gamble with death*. Englewood Cliffs: Prentice-Hall, 1971.

Li, F. Suicide among chemists. *Archives of Environmental Health*, 1969, 19, 518–520.

Liberman, R., and Eckman, T. Behavior therapy versus insight-oriented therapy for repeated suicide attempters. *Archives of General Psychiatry*, 1981, 38, 1126–1130.

Linden, L., and Hale, B. The choice of suicidal methods. In R. Litman (ed.). *Proceedings of the 6th International Conference for Suicide Prevention*. Ann Arbor: Edwards, 1972, 165–170.

Lippman, S. N. Kelly v. R.G. Industries. *Tort and Insurance Law Journal*, 1986, 21, 493–508.

Low, A.A., Farmer, R.D.T., Jones, D.R., and Rohde, J.R. Suicide in England and Wales. *Psychological Medicine*, 1981, 11, 359–368.

McDonald, J. *The girl in the plain brown wrapper*. Greenwich, CT: Fawcett, 1968.

Malleson, A. Suicide prevention: A myth or a mandate? *British Journal of Psychiatry*, 1973, 122, 238–239; 123, 612–613.

Maniam, T. Suicide and parasuicide in a hill resort in Malaysia. *British Journal of Psychiatry*, 1988, 153, 222–225.

Marks, A. Sex differences and their effect upon cultural evaluations of methods of self-destruction. *Omega*, 1977, 8, 65–70.

Marks, A., and Abernathy, T. Towards a sociocultural perspective on means of self destruction. *Life-Threatening Behavior*, 1974, 4, 3–17.

Marks, A., and Stokes, C. Socialization, firearms and suicide. *Social Problems*, 1976, 23, 622–629.

Markush, R.E., and Bartolucci, A. Firearms and suicide in the United States. *American Journal of Public Health*, 1984, 74, 123–127.

Martin, M.J., Hunt, T.K., and Hulley, S.B. The cost of hospitalization for firearm injuries. *Journal of the American Medical Association*, 1988, 260, 3048–3050.

McDowall, D., and Loftin, C. Collective security and fatal firearm accidents. *Criminology*, 1985, 23, 401–416.

McMurray, J.J., Northbridge, D.B., Abernethy, V.A., and Lawson, A.A.M. The trends in self-poisoning in West-Fife. *Quarterly Journal of Medicine*, 1987, New Series 65, 835–843.

McWilliams, C. Suicide bridge. *Pacific Weekly*, 1936, 6, 362–365.

Medoff, M.H., and Magaddino, J.P. Suicides and firearm control laws. *Evaluation Review*, 1983, 7, 357–372.

Miller, H., Coombs, D., Leeper, J., and Barton, S. An analysis of the effects of suicide prevention facilities on suicide rates in the US. *American Journal of Public Health*, 1984, 74, 340–343.

Montgomery, S., and Montgomery, D. Drug treatment of suicidal behavior. *Advances in Biochemistry and Psychopharmacology*, 1982, 32, 347–355.

Montgomery, S., and Montgomery, D. Drug treatment of suicidal behavior. *Advances in Biochemistry and Psychopharmacology*, 1984, 39, 315–317.

Morton, F. *Report of the enquiry into the safety of natural gas as a fuel*. London: Her Majesty's Stationery Office, 1970.

Moss, R.J. The big leap: On-site prevention. *Psychology Today*, August 1986, 14.

Murray, D.R. Handguns, gun control laws and firearm violence. *Social Problems*, 1975, 23, 81–92.

Newton, G., and Zimring, F. *Firearms and violence in American life*. Washington, DC: U.S. Government Printing Office, 1969.

Noomen, P. Suicide in the Netherlands. In N. L. Farberow (ed.). *Suicide in different cultures*. Baltimore: University Park Press, 1975.

Oast, S.P., and Zitrin, A. A public health approach to suicide prevention. *American Journal of Public Health*, 1974, 65, 144–147.

Oliver, R.G., and Hetzel, B.S. Rise and fall of suicide rates in Australia: Relation to sedative availability. *Medical Journal of Australia*, 1972, 2, 919–923.

Oliver, R.G., and Hetzel, B. S. An analysis of recent trends in suicide in Australia. *International Journal of Epidemiology*, 1973, 2, 91–101.

Orr, L.D. The effectiveness of automobile safety regulation. *American Journal of Public Health*, 1984, 74, 1384–1389.

Patel, N.S. Pathology of suicide. *Medicine, Science and Law*, 1973, 13, 103–109.

Paykel, E. Life stress. In L. Hankoff and B. Einsidler (eds.). *Suicide*. Littleton, MA: PSG, 1979, 225–234.

Peebles. M.W.H. *Evolution of the gas industry*. London: Macmillan, 1980.

Phillips, D.P. The influence of suggestion on suicide. *American Sociological Review*, 1974, 39, 340–354.

Phillips, D.P., and Carstensen, L.L. The effect of suicide stories on various demographic groups 1968–1985. *Suicide and Life-Threatening Behavior*, 1988, 18, 100–113.

Poore, A.C.G. Packaging: Can it help to reduce the incidence of poisoning? *Journal of International Medical Research*, 1976, 4 (Suppl 4) 76–96.

Quinn, B., Anderson, H., Bradley, M., Goetting, P., and Shriver, P. *Churches and church membership in the United States*. Atlantic: Glenmary Research Center, 1982.

Rao, A.V. Suicide in India. In N.L. Farberow (ed.). *Suicide in different cultures*. Baltimore: University Park Press, 1975.

Ratcliffe, R.W. The open door. *Lancet*, 1962, ii, 188–190.

Registrar General. *The Registrar-General's statistical review of England and Wales. Part. 1, Medical*. London: Her Majesty's Stationery Office, 1961.

Reppetto, T.A. Crime prevention and the displacement phenomonen. *Crime and Delinquency*, 1976, 22, 166–177.

Resnick, H., and Hathorne, B. *Suicide prevention in the 70s*. Rockville: National Institute of Mental Health, 1973.

Rin, H. Suicide in Taiwan. In N.L. Farberow (ed.). *Suicide in different cultures*. Baltimore: University Park Press, 1975.

Robin, A.A., and Freeman-Browne, D. Drugs left at home by psychiatric patients. *British Medical Journal*, 1968, 3, 424–425.

Rosen, D.H. Suicide survivors: A follow-up study of persons who survived jumping from the Golden Gate and San Francisco–Oakland Bay Bridges *Western Journal of Medicine*, 1975, 122, 289–294.

Ross, O., and Kreitman, N. A further investigation of differences in the suicide rates of England and Wales and Scotland. *British Journal of Psychiatry*, 1975, 127, 575–582.

Rudestam, K., and Imbroll, D. Societal reaction to a child's death by suicide. *Journal of Consulting & Clinical Psychology*, 1983, 51, 461–462.

Sainsbury, P. The validity and reliability of trends in suicide rates. *Quarterly Statistics of the World Health Organization*, 1983, 36, 339–345.

Sainsbury, P. The epidemiology of suicide. In A. Roy (ed.). *Suicide*. Baltimore: Williams & Wilkins, 1986.

Sainsbury, P., Jenkins, J., and Levey, A. The social correlates of suicide in Europe. In R. Farmer and S. Hirsch (eds.). *The suicide syndrome*. London: Croom Helm, 1980.

Seiden, R.H. Suicide capital? A study of the San Franciso suicide rate, *Bulletin of Suicidology*, 1967, 2, 1–10.

Seiden, R.H. Suicide prevention: A public health/public policy approach. *Omega*, 1977, 8, 267–276.

Seiden, R.H., and Spence, M. A tale of two bridges. *Omega*, 1983–1984, 201–209.

Seitz, S.T. Firearms, homicides and gun control effectiveness. *Law and Society Review*, 1972, 6, 595–613.

Shneidman, E.S. *Definition of suicide*. New York: Wiley–Interscience, 1985.

Siegel, R., and Siegel, L, Use of barbiturate suppositories. *Western Journal of Medicine*, 1981, 135, 160.

Sim, N. Gun control and suicide. *Proceedings of the 10th International Congress for Suicide Prevention*. Ottawa: IASP, 1979, 187–189.

Smith, A.O. The manufacture and distribution of handguns as an abnormally dangerous activity. *The University of Chicago Law Review*, 1987, 54, 369–406.

Stack, S. Relgion and suicide. *Social Psychiatry*, 1980, 15, 65–70.

Stack, S. Celebrities and suicide. *American Sociological Review*, 1987, 52, 401–412.

Stengel, E. *Suicide and attempted suicide*. Baltimore: Penguin, 1964.

Stoller, A. Suicides and attempted suicides in Australia. *Proceedings of the 5th. International Conference on Suicide Prevention*. London, 1969.

Taylor, M.C., and Wicks, J.W. The choice of weapons: A study of methods of suicide by sex, race, and religion. *Suicide and Life-Threatening Behavior*, 1980, 10, 142–149.

Taylor, S. *Durkheim and the study of suicide*. London: Macmillan, 1982.

Thorson, J., Svenson, L., and Nilsson, J. Carbon monoxide poisoning and cars. On modification of opportunities for Suicide. *AAAM*, 32rd Annual Conference, Seattle, 1988.

Tonso, W.R. *Gun and society*. Washington, DC: University Press of America, 1982.

Uhlenberg, P., and Eggebeen, D. The declining well-being of American adolescents. *Public Interest*, 1986, 82, 25–38.

U.S. Census Bureau. *Statistical Abstract of the United States, 1984*. Washington, DC: U.S. Government Printing Office, 1984.

Velkoff, M.S., and Huberty, T.J. Thinking patterns and motivation. In D. Capuzzi and L. Golden (eds.) *Preventing adolescent suicide*. Munde, IN: Accelerated Development, 1988.

Walk, D. Suicide and community care. *British Journal of Psychiatry*, 1967, 113, 1381–1391.

Weissman, M.M. The epidemiology of suicide attempts, 1960–1971. *Archives of General Psychiatry*, 1974, 30, 737–746.

Wells, N. *Suicide and deliberate self-harm*. London: Office of Health Economics, 1981.

Welu, T.C. Broadening the focus of suicide prevention activities utilizing the public health model. *American Journal of Public Health*, 1972, 62, 1625–1628.

Westermeyer, J. (editorial). Firearms, legislation, and suicide prevention. *American Journal of Public Health*, 1984, 74, 108.

White-Bowden, S. *Everything to live for*. New York: Poseidon 1985.

Whitlock, F.A. Suicide in Brisbane, 1956 to 1973. *Medical Journal of Australia*, 1975, 1, 737–743.

Wilde, G.J.S. Beyond the concept of risk homeostasis. *Accident Analysis and Prevention*, 1986, 18, 377–401.

Williams, T.I. *A history of the British gas industry*. New York: Oxford University Press, 1981.

Winslow, C.E.A. *The evolution and significance of the modern public health campaign*. New Haven: Yale University Press, 1923.

Wintemute, G.J., Teret, S.P., Krauss, J.F., and Wright, M.W. The choice of weapons in firearm suicides. *American Journal of Public Health*. 1988, 78, 824–826.

Wold, C., and Litman, R.E. Suicide after contact with a suicide prevention center. *Archives of General Psychiatry*, 1973, 28, 735–739.

World Health Organization. *International Classification of Diseases*, Geneva: WHO, 1967.

World Health Organization. *Changing patterns in suicide behavior*. European Reports and Studies No. 74, Copenhagen: WHO, 1982.

Wright, J.D., Rossi, P.H., and Daly, K. *Under the gun*. New York: Aldine, 1983.

Yamasawa, K., Nishimukai, H., Ohbora, Y., and Inoue, K. Statistical study of suicides through intoxification. *Acta Medicinae Legalis et Socialis*, 1980, 30, 187–192.

Zimring, F. Firearms and federal law. *Journal of Legal Studies*, 1975, 4, 133–198.

Zimring, F.E., and Hawkins, G. *The citizen's guide to gun control*. New York: Macmillan, 1987.

Index